FREE
GMP / QMS
Webinar Training
Satisfy your Annual GMP Training Requirement

Sponsored by:

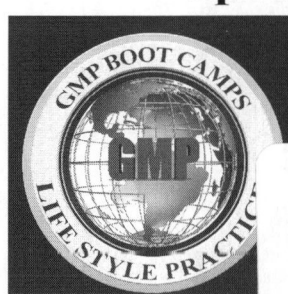

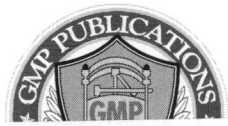

AF275305

Conducted Monthly
Sign-up at:

www.fda.com

or

www.gmpbootcamps.com

The Code of Federal Regulations
Title 21 – Food and Drugs

Part 11
ELECTRONIC RECORDS; ELECTRONIC SIGNATURES

Part 58
GOOD LABORATORY PRACTICE FOR NON CLINICAL LABORATORY STUDIES

Parts 210 & 211
cGMP IN MANUFACTURING, PROCESSING, PACKING, OR HOLDING OF DRUGS AND FINISHED PHARMACEUTICALS

Part 600
BIOLOGICAL PRODUCTS: GENERAL

Part 601
LICENSING

Part 610
GENERAL BIOLOGICAL PRODUCTS STANDARDS

Part 820
QUALITY SYSTEM REGULATION

Printed by GMP Publications, Inc.
Tel: 866-544-9007 or 856-810-7331
Fax: 866-544-9002
http://www.gmppublications.com
sales@gmppublications.com

FDA.COM
On-Line Information Portal
& Discussion Groups

FDA.COM is an internet communications site dedicated to supporting the regulated industry by providing a free on-line portal, focusing on the mutual sharing of professional and Government Food, Drug and Regulated information through interactive topic specific discussion groups, online databases and instant access.

FDA.COM is the 'next step', taking industry professionals and visitors beyond The Food and Drug Administration Department. Where the Food and Drug Administration provides the regulations that creates the Laws that Pharmaceuticals, Biotechnology and other Regulated Industry must abide to, they lack in providing a forum of discussing or guiding the industry as to the 'How' and 'Why' to comply.

Every day, thousands of industry professionals come to FDA.COM to find guidance. FDA.COM delivers immediate streamlined quality information to the industry professionals by industry leaders.

Discussion Groups and Open Forums

Food & Drug Administration Links
GMP, GLP, GCP Assistance
Seminars and Conference Listings
Regulatory Guidance
Databases Archives
Guidance Documents Repository
Global Market Place
Classified
e-Newsletters
Templates and Forms Repository
Career Centers and Resume Banks
Advertising Assistance and Promotions

Become a FDA.COM Sponsor today. Sponsors are Industry Leaders, Vendors, Contractors or Professional Service firms, who would field technical and compliance issues by the industry. Sponsors currently enjoy the exclusivity of sponsoring their field or technology sector, and by assisting the industry, enables those Sponsors to stand out as the authoritarian leaders of their specific industry. And at the same time allowing industry leaders to promote their services and products!

Marketing your products or services? With over 2,000,000 visitors a month, FDA.COM is the world's premier global regulatory information resource.

FDA.COM
866-544-9001
Fax 866-544-9002
info@fda.com

The Code of Federal Regulations
Title 21 – Food and Drugs

Part 11
ELECTRONIC RECORDS;
ELECTRONIC SIGNATURES

GUIDANCE FOR INDUSTRY
PART 11
SCOPE AND APPLICATION
August 2003

Printed by GMP Publications, Inc.
Tel: 866-544-9007 or 856-810-7331
Fax: 866-544-9002
http://www.gmppublications.com
sales@gmppublications.com

PART 11--ELECTRONIC RECORDS; ELECTRONIC SIGNATURES

Subpart A--General Provisions

Subpart B--Electronic Records

Subpart C--Electronic Signatures

Authority: 21 U.S.C. 321-393; 42 U.S.C. 262.

Source: 62 FR 13464, Mar. 20, 1997, unless otherwise noted.

Subpart A--General Provisions

§11.1   Scope.

(a) The regulations in this part set forth the criteria under which the agency considers electronic records, electronic signatures, and handwritten signatures executed to electronic records to be trustworthy, reliable, and generally equivalent to paper records and handwritten signatures executed on paper.

(b) This part applies to records in electronic form that are created, modified, maintained, archived, retrieved, or transmitted, under any records requirements set forth in agency regulations. This part also applies to electronic records submitted to the agency under requirements of the Federal Food, Drug, and Cosmetic Act and the Public Health Service Act, even if such records are not specifically identified in agency regulations. However, this part does not apply to paper records that are, or have been, transmitted by electronic means.

(c) Where electronic signatures and their associated electronic records meet the requirements of this part, the agency will consider the electronic signatures to be equivalent to full handwritten signatures, initials, and other general signings as required by agency regulations, unless specifically excepted by regulation(s) effective on or after August 20, 1997.

(d) Electronic records that meet the requirements of this part may be used in lieu of paper records, in accordance with §11.2, unless paper records are specifically required.

(e) Computer systems (including hardware and software), controls, and attendant documentation maintained under this part shall be readily available for, and subject to, FDA inspection.

(f) This part does not apply to records required to be established or maintained by §§1.326 through 1.368 of this chapter. Records that satisfy the requirements of part 1, subpart J of this chapter, but that also are required under other applicable statutory provisions or regulations, remain subject to this part.

(g) This part does not apply to electronic signatures obtained under §101.11(d) of this chapter.

(h) This part does not apply to electronic signatures obtained under §101.8(d) of this chapter.

(i) This part does not apply to records required to be established or maintained by part 117 of this chapter. Records that satisfy the requirements of part 117 of this chapter, but that also are required under other applicable statutory provisions or regulations, remain subject to this part.

(j) This part does not apply to records required to be established or maintained by part 507 of this chapter. Records that satisfy the requirements of part 507 of this chapter, but that also are required under other applicable statutory provisions or regulations, remain subject to this part.

(k) This part does not apply to records required to be established or maintained by part 112 of this chapter. Records that satisfy the requirements of part 112 of this chapter, but that also are required under other applicable statutory provisions or regulations, remain subject to this part.

(l) This part does not apply to records required to be established or maintained by subpart L of part 1 of this chapter. Records that satisfy the requirements of subpart L of part 1 of this chapter, but that also are required under other applicable statutory provisions or regulations, remain subject to this part.

(m) This part does not apply to records required to be established or maintained by subpart M of part 1 of this chapter. Records that satisfy the requirements of subpart M of part 1 of this chapter, but that also are required under other applicable statutory provisions or regulations, remain subject to this part.

(n) This part does not apply to records required to be established or maintained by subpart O of part 1 of this chapter. Records that satisfy the requirements of subpart O of part 1 of this chapter, but that also are required under other applicable statutory provisions or regulations, remain subject to this part.

(o) This part does not apply to records required to be established or maintained by part 121 of this chapter. Records that satisfy the requirements of part 121 of this chapter, but that also are required under other applicable statutory provisions or regulations, remain subject to this part.

(p) This part does not apply to records required to be established or maintained by subpart R of part 1 of this chapter. Records that satisfy the requirements of subpart R of part 1 of this chapter, but that also are required under other applicable statutory provisions or regulations, remain subject to this part.

[62 FR 13464, Mar. 20, 1997, as amended at 69 FR 71655, Dec. 9, 2004; 79 FR 71253, Dec. 1, 2014; 80 FR 71253, June 19, 2015; 80 FR 56144, 56336, Sept. 17, 2015; 80 FR 74352, 74547, 74667, Nov. 27, 2015; 81 FR 20170, Apr. 6, 2016; 81 FR 34218, May 27, 2016; 86 FR 68839, Feb. 1, 2022]

§11.2　　Implementation.

(a) For records required to be maintained but not submitted to the agency, persons may use electronic records in lieu of paper records or electronic signatures in lieu of traditional signatures, in whole or in part, provided that the requirements of this part are met.

(b) For records submitted to the agency, persons may use electronic records in lieu of paper records or electronic signatures in lieu of traditional signatures, in whole or in part, provided that:

(1) The requirements of this part are met; and

(2) The document or parts of a document to be submitted have been identified in public docket No. 92S-0251 as being the type of submission the agency accepts in electronic form. This docket will identify specifically what types of documents or parts of documents are acceptable for submission in electronic form without paper records and the agency receiving unit(s) (e.g., specific center, office, division, branch) to which such submissions may be made. Documents to agency receiving unit(s) not specified in the public docket will not be considered as official if they are submitted in electronic form; paper forms of such

documents will be considered as official and must accompany any electronic records. Persons are expected to consult with the intended agency receiving unit for details on how (e.g., method of transmission, media, file formats, and technical protocols) and whether to proceed with the electronic submission.

§11.3   Definitions.

(a) The definitions and interpretations of terms contained in section 201 of the act apply to those terms when used in this part.

(b) The following definitions of terms also apply to this part:

(1) *Act* means the Federal Food, Drug, and Cosmetic Act (§201-903 (21 U.S.C. 321-393)).

(2) *Agency* means the Food and Drug Administration.

(3) *Biometrics* means a method of verifying an individual's identity based on measurement of the individual's physical feature(s) or repeatable action(s) where those features and/or actions are both unique to that individual and measurable.

(4) *Closed system* means an environment in which system access is controlled by persons who are responsible for the content of electronic records that are on the system.

(5) *Digital signature* means an electronic signature based upon cryptographic methods of originator authentication, computed by using a set of rules and a set of parameters such that the identity of the signer and the integrity of the data can be verified.

(6) *Electronic record* means any combination of text, graphics, data, audio, pictorial, or other information representation in digital form that is created, modified, maintained, archived, retrieved, or distributed by a computer system.

(7) *Electronic signature* means a computer data compilation of any symbol or series of symbols executed, adopted, or authorized by an individual to be the legally binding equivalent of the individual's handwritten signature.

(8) *Handwritten signature* means the scripted name or legal mark of an individual handwritten by that individual and executed or adopted with the present intention to authenticate a writing in a permanent form. The act of signing with a writing or marking instrument such as a pen or stylus is preserved. The scripted name or legal mark, while conventionally applied to paper, may also be applied to other devices that capture the name or mark.

(9) *Open system* means an environment in which system access is not controlled by persons who are responsible for the content of electronic records that are on the system.

Subpart B--Electronic Records
§11.10 Controls for closed systems.

Persons who use closed systems to create, modify, maintain, or transmit electronic records shall employ procedures and controls designed to ensure the authenticity, integrity, and, when appropriate, the confidentiality of electronic records, and to ensure that the signer cannot readily repudiate the signed record as not genuine. Such procedures and controls shall include the following:

(a) Validation of systems to ensure accuracy, reliability, consistent intended performance, and the ability to discern invalid or altered records.

(b) The ability to generate accurate and complete copies of records in both human readable and electronic form suitable for inspection, review, and copying by the agency. Persons should contact the agency if there are any questions regarding the ability of the agency to perform such review and copying of the electronic records.

(c) Protection of records to enable their accurate and ready retrieval throughout the records retention period.

(d) Limiting system access to authorized individuals.

(e) Use of secure, computer-generated, time-stamped audit trails to independently record the date and time of operator entries and actions that create, modify, or delete electronic records. Record changes shall not obscure previously recorded information. Such audit trail documentation shall be retained for a period at least as long as that required for the subject electronic records and shall be available for agency review and copying.

(f) Use of operational system checks to enforce permitted sequencing of steps and events, as appropriate.

(g) Use of authority checks to ensure that only authorized individuals can use the system, electronically sign a record, access the operation or computer system input or output device, alter a record, or perform the operation at hand.

(h) Use of device (e.g., terminal) checks to determine, as appropriate, the validity of the source of data input or operational instruction.

(i) Determination that persons who develop, maintain, or use electronic record/electronic signature systems have the education, training, and experience to perform their assigned tasks.

(j) The establishment of, and adherence to, written policies that hold individuals accountable and responsible for actions initiated under their electronic signatures, in order to deter record and signature falsification.

(k) Use of appropriate controls over systems documentation including:

(1) Adequate controls over the distribution of, access to, and use of documentation for system operation and maintenance.

(2) Revision and change control procedures to maintain an audit trail that documents time-sequenced development and modification of systems documentation.

§11.30   Controls for open systems.

Persons who use open systems to create, modify, maintain, or transmit electronic records shall employ procedures and controls designed to ensure the authenticity, integrity, and, as appropriate, the confidentiality of electronic records from the point of their creation to the point of their receipt. Such procedures and controls shall include those identified in §11.10, as appropriate, and additional measures such as document encryption and use of appropriate digital signature standards to ensure, as necessary under the circumstances, record authenticity, integrity, and confidentiality.

§11.50   Signature manifestations.

(a) Signed electronic records shall contain information associated with the signing that clearly indicates all of the following:
(1) The printed name of the signer;
(2) The date and time when the signature was executed; and
(3) The meaning (such as review, approval, responsibility, or authorship) associated with the signature.
(b) The items identified in paragraphs (a)(1), (a)(2), and (a)(3) of this section shall be subject to the same controls as for electronic records and shall be included as part of any human readable form of the electronic record (such as electronic display or printout).

§11.70   Signature/record linking.

Electronic signatures and handwritten signatures executed to electronic records shall be linked to their respective electronic records to ensure that the signatures cannot be excised, copied, or otherwise transferred to falsify an electronic record by ordinary means.

Subpart C--Electronic Signatures
§11.100   General requirements.

(a) Each electronic signature shall be unique to one individual and shall not be reused by, or reassigned to, anyone else.
(b) Before an organization establishes, assigns, certifies, or otherwise sanctions an individual's electronic signature, or any element of such electronic signature, the organization shall verify the identity of the individual.
(c) Persons using electronic signatures shall, prior to or

at the time of such use, certify to the agency that the electronic signatures in their system, used on or after August 20, 1997, are intended to be the legally binding equivalent of traditional handwritten signatures.

(1) The certification shall be submitted in paper form and signed with a traditional handwritten signature, to the Office of Regional Operations (HFC-100), 5600 Fishers Lane, Rockville, MD 20857.

(2) Persons using electronic signatures shall, upon agency request, provide additional certification or testimony that a specific electronic signature is the legally binding equivalent of the signer's handwritten signature.

§11.200　Electronic signature components and controls.

(a) Electronic signatures that are not based upon biometrics shall:

(1) Employ at least two distinct identification components such as an identification code and password.

(i) When an individual executes a series of signings during a single, continuous period of controlled system access, the first signing shall be executed using all electronic signature components; subsequent signings shall be executed using at least one electronic signature component that is only executable by, and designed to be used only by, the individual.

(ii) When an individual executes one or more signings not performed during a single, continuous period of controlled system access, each signing shall be executed using all of the electronic signature components.

(2) Be used only by their genuine owners; and

(3) Be administered and executed to ensure that attempted use of an individual's electronic signature by anyone other than its genuine owner requires collaboration of two or more individuals.

(b) Electronic signatures based upon biometrics shall be designed to ensure that they cannot be used by anyone other than their genuine owners.

§11.300 Controls for identification codes/passwords.

Persons who use electronic signatures based upon use of identification codes in combination with passwords shall employ controls to ensure their security and integrity. Such controls shall include:

(a) Maintaining the uniqueness of each combined identification code and password, such that no two individuals have the same combination of identification code and password.

(b) Ensuring that identification code and password issuances are periodically checked, recalled, or revised (e.g., to cover such events as password aging).

(c) Following loss management procedures to electronically deauthorize lost, stolen, missing, or otherwise potentially compromised tokens, cards, and other devices that bear or generate identification code or password information, and to issue temporary or permanent replacements using suitable, rigorous controls.

(d) Use of transaction safeguards to prevent unauthorized use of passwords and/or identification codes, and to detect and report in an immediate and urgent manner any attempts at their unauthorized use to the system security unit, and, as appropriate, to organizational management.

(e) Initial and periodic testing of devices, such as tokens or cards, that bear or generate identification code or password information to ensure that they function properly and have not been altered in an unauthorized manner.

Notes

Guidance for Industry
Part 11, Electronic Records;
Electronic Signatures — Scope and Application

Office of Training and Communications
Division of Drug Information
Center for Drug Evaluation and Research (CDER)
WO51, Room 2201
10903 New Hampshire Ave
Silver Spring, MD 20993
Phone: 301-796-3400 Fax: 301-847-8714
E-mail: druginfo@fda.hhs.gov
http://www.fda.gov/Drugs/GuidanceComplianceRegulatoryI
nformation/Guidances/default.htm

or

Office of Communication, Training and
Manufacturers Assistance, HFM-40
Center for Biologics Evaluation and Research (CBER)
Phone: the Voice Information System at
800-835-4709 or 301-827-1800
http://www.fda.gov/BiologicsBloodVaccines/GuidanceComp
lianceRegulatoryInformation/Guidances/default.htm

or

Communications Staff (HFV-12),
Center for Veterinary Medicine (CVM)
(Tel) 240-276-9300
http://www.fda.gov/AnimalVeterinary/GuidanceCompliance
Enforcement/GuidanceforIndustry/default.htm

or

Division of Small Manufacturers, International, and
Consumer Assistance (HFZ-220)
http://www.fda.gov/cdrh/ggpmain.html
Manufacturers Assistance Phone Number: 800-638-2041
or 301-796-7100

or

Center for Food Safety and Applied Nutrition (CFSAN)
http://www.fda.gov/Food/GuidanceRegulation/Guidance
DocumentsRegulatoryInformation/default.htm

U.S. Department of Health and Human Services
Food and Drug Administration
Center for Drug Evaluation and Research (CDER)
Center for Biologics Evaluation and Research (CBER)
Center for Devices and Radiological Health (CDRH)
Center for Food Safety and Applied Nutrition (CFSAN)
Center for Veterinary Medicine (CVM)
Office of Regulatory Affairs (ORA)

August 2003
Pharmaceutical CGMPs

TABLE OF CONTENTS

Guidance for Industry[1]
Part 11, Electronic Records; Electronic Signatures Scope and Application
Contains Nonbinding RecommendationsM

This guidance represents the Food and Drug Administration's (FDA's) current thinking on this topic. It does not create or confer any rights for or on any person and does not operate to bind FDA or the public. You can use an alternative approach if the approach satisfies the requirements of the applicable statutes and regulations. If you want to discuss an alternative approach, contact the FDA staff responsible for implementing this guidance. If you cannot identify the appropriate FDA staff, call the appropriate number listed on the title page of this guidance.

I. INTRODUCTION

This guidance is intended to describe the Food and Drug Administration's (FDA's) current thinking regarding the scope and application of part 11 of Title 21 of the Code of Federal Regulations; Electronic Records; Electronic Signatures (21 CFR Part 11).[2]

This document provides guidance to persons who, in fulfillment of a requirement in a statute or another part of FDA's regulations to maintain records or submit information to FDA[3], have chosen to maintain the records or submit designated information electronically and, as a result, have become subject to part 11. Part 11 applies to records in electronic form that are created, modified, maintained, archived, retrieved, or transmitted under any records requirements set forth in Agency regulations. Part 11 also applies to electronic records submitted to the Agency under the Federal Food, Drug, and Cosmetic Act (the Act) and the Public Health Service Act (the PHS Act), even if such records are not specifically identified in Agency regulations (§ 11.1). The underlying requirements set forth in the Act, PHS Act, and FDA regulations (other than part 11) are referred to in this guidance document as *predicate rules*.

As an outgrowth of its current good manufacturing practice (CGMP) initiative for human and animal drugs and biologics,[4] FDA is re-examining part 11 as it applies to all FDA regulated products. We anticipate initiating rulemaking to change part 11 as a result of that re-examination. This guidance explains that we will narrowly interpret the scope of part 11. While the re-examination of part 11 is under way, we intend to exercise enforcement discretion with respect to certain part 11 requirements. That is, we do not intend to take enforcement action to enforce compliance with the validation, audit trail, record retention, and record copying requirements of part 11 as explained in this guidance. However, records must still be maintained or submitted in accordance with the underlying predicate rules, and the Agency can take regulatory action for noncompliance with such predicate rules.

In addition, we intend to exercise enforcement discretion and do not intend to take (or recommend) action to enforce any part 11 requirements with regard to systems that were operational before August 20, 1997, the effective date of part 11 (commonly known as legacy systems) under the circumstances described in section III.C.3 of this guidance.

Note that part 11 remains in effect and that this exercise of enforcement discretion applies only as identified in this guidance.

FDA's guidance documents, including this guidance, do not establish legally enforceable responsibilities. Instead, guidances describe the Agency's current thinking on a topic and should be viewed only as recommendations, unless specific regulatory or statutory requirements are cited. The use of the word should in Agency guidances means that something is suggested or recommended, but not required.

II. BACKGROUND

In March of 1997, FDA issued final part 11 regulations that provide criteria for acceptance by FDA, under certain circumstances, of electronic records, electronic signatures, and handwritten signatures executed to electronic records as equivalent to paper records and handwritten signatures executed on paper. These regulations, which apply to all FDA program areas, were intended to permit the widest possible use of electronic technology, compatible with FDA's responsibility to protect the public health.

After part 11 became effective in August 1997, significant discussions ensued among industry, contractors, and the Agency concerning the interpretation and implementation of the regulations. FDA has (1) spoken about part 11 at many conferences and met numerous times with an industry coalition and other interested parties in an effort to hear more about potential part 11 issues; (2) published a compliance policy guide, CPG 7153.17: Enforcement Policy: 21 CFR Part 11; Electronic Records; Electronic Signatures; and (3) published numerous draft guidance documents including the following:

• *21 CFR Part 11; Electronic Records; Electronic Signatures, Validation*

• *21 CFR Part 11; Electronic Records; Electronic Signatures, Glossary of Terms*

• *21 CFR Part 11; Electronic Records; Electronic Signatures, Time Stamps*

• *21 CFR Part 11; Electronic Records; Electronic Signatures, Maintenance of Electronic Records*

• *21 CFR Part 11; Electronic Records; Electronic Signatures, Electronic Copies of Electronic Records*

Throughout all of these communications, concerns have been raised that some interpretations of the part 11 requirements would (1) unnecessarily restrict the use of electronic technology in a manner that is inconsistent with FDA's stated intent in issuing the rule, (2) significantly increase the costs of compliance to an extent that was not contemplated at the time the rule was drafted, and (3) discourage innovation and technological advances without providing a significant public health benefit. These concerns have been raised particularly in the areas of part 11 requirements for validation, audit trails, record retention, record copying, and legacy systems.

As a result of these concerns, we decided to review the part 11 documents and related issues, particularly in light of the Agency's CGMP initiative. In the *Federal Register* of February 4, 2003 (68 FR 5645), we announced the withdrawal of the draft guidance for industry, *21 CFR Part 11; Electronic Records; Electronic Signatures, Electronic Copies of Electronic Records.* We had decided we wanted to minimize industry time spent reviewing and commenting on the draft guidance when that draft guidance may no longer represent our approach under the CGMP initiative. Then, in the *Federal Register* of February 25, 2003 (68 FR 8775), we announced the withdrawal of the part 11 draft guidance documents on validation, glossary of terms, time stamps,[5] maintenance of electronic records, and CPG 7153.17. We received valuable public comments on these draft guidances, and we plan to use that information to help with future decision-making with respect to part 11. We do not intend to re-issue these draft guidance documents or the CPG.

We are now re-examining part 11, and we anticipate initiating rulemaking to revise provisions of that regulation. To avoid unnecessary resource expenditures to comply with part 11 requirements, we are issuing this guidance to describe how we intend to exercise enforcement discretion with regard to certain part 11 requirements during the re-examination of part 11. As mentioned previously, part 11 remains in effect during this re-examination period.

III. DISCUSSION

A. Overall Approach to Part 11 Requirements

As described in more detail below, the approach outlined in this guidance is based on three main elements:

• Part 11 will be interpreted narrowly; we are now clarifying that fewer records will be considered subject to part 11.

• For those records that remain subject to part 11, we intend to exercise enforcement discretion with regard to part 11 requirements for validation, audit trails, record retention, and record copying in the manner described in this guidance and with regard to all part 11 requirements for systems that were operational before the effective date of part 11 (also known as legacy systems).

• We will enforce all predicate rule requirements, including predicate rule record and recordkeeping requirements.

It is important to note that FDA's exercise of enforcement discretion as described in this guidance is limited to specified part 11 requirements (setting aside legacy systems, as to which the extent of enforcement discretion, under certain circumstances, will be more broad). We intend to enforce all other provisions of part 11 including, but not limited to, certain controls for closed systems in §11.10. For example, we intend to enforce provisions related to the following controls and requirements:

• limiting system access to authorized individuals
• use of operational system checks
• use of authority checks
• use of device checks

• determination that persons who develop, maintain, or use electronic systems have the education, training, and experience to perform their assigned tasks

• establishment of and adherence to written policies that hold individuals accountable for actions initiated under their electronic signatures

• appropriate controls over systems documentation

• controls for open systems corresponding to controls for closed systems bulleted above (§ 11.30)

• requirements related to electronic signatures (e.g., §§11.50, 11.70, 11.100, 11.200, and 11.300)

We expect continued compliance with these provisions, and we will continue to enforce them. Furthermore, persons must comply with applicable predicate rules, and records that are required to be maintained or submitted must remain secure and reliable in accordance with the predicate rules.

B. Details of Approach – Scope of Part 11

1. Narrow Interpretation of Scope

We understand that there is some confusion about the scope of part 11. Some have understood the scope of part 11 to be very broad. We believe that some of those broad interpretations could lead to unnecessary controls and costs and could discourage innovation and technological advances without providing added benefit to the public health. As a result, we want to clarify that the Agency intends to interpret the scope of part 11 narrowly.

Under the narrow interpretation of the scope of part 11, with respect to records required to be maintained under predicate rules or submitted to FDA, when persons choose to use records in electronic format in place of paper format, part 11 would apply. On the other hand, when persons use computers to generate paper printouts of electronic records, and those paper records meet all the requirements of the applicable predicate rules and persons rely on the paper records to perform their regulated activities, FDA would generally not consider persons to be "using electronic records in lieu of paper records" under §§11.2(a) and 11.2(b). In these instances, the use of computer systems in the generation of paper records would not trigger part 11.

2. Definition of Part 11 Records

Under this narrow interpretation, FDA considers part 11 to be applicable to the following records or signatures in electronic format (part 11 records or signatures):

• Records that are required to be maintained under predicate rule requirements and that are maintained in electronic format *in place of paper format.* On the other hand, records (and any associated signatures) that are not required to be retained under predicate rules, but that are nonetheless maintained in electronic format, are not part 11 records.

We recommend that you determine, based on the predicate rules, whether specific records are part 11 records. We recommend that you document such decisions.

• Records that are required to be maintained under predicate rules, that are maintained in electronic format *in addition to paper format,* and that *are relied on to perform regulated activities.*

In some cases, actual business practices may dictate whether you are *using* electronic records instead of paper records under §11.2(a). For example, if a record is required to be maintained under a predicate rule and you use a computer to generate a paper printout of the electronic records, but you nonetheless rely on the electronic record to perform regulated activities, the Agency may consider you to be using the electronic record instead of the paper record. That is, the Agency may take your business practices into account in determining whether part 11 applies.

Accordingly, we recommend that, for each record required to be maintained under predicate rules, you determine in advance whether you plan to rely on the electronic record or paper record to perform regulated activities. We recommend that you document this decision (e.g., in a Standard Operating Procedure (SOP), or specification document).

• Records submitted to FDA, under predicate rules (even if such records are not specifically identified in Agency regulations) in electronic format (assuming the records have been identified in docket number 92S-0251 as the types of submissions the Agency accepts in electronic format). However, a record that is not itself submitted, but is used in generating a submission, is not a part 11 record unless it is otherwise required to be maintained under a predicate rule and it is maintained in electronic format.

• Electronic signatures that are intended to be the equivalent of handwritten signatures, initials, and other general signings required by predicate rules. Part 11 signatures include electronic signatures that are used, for example, to document the fact that certain events or actions occurred in accordance with the predicate rule (e.g. *approved, reviewed,* and *verified*).

C. Approach to Specific Part 11 Requirements

1. Validation

The Agency intends to exercise enforcement discretion regarding specific part 11 requirements for validation of computerized systems (§11.10(a) and corresponding requirements in §11.30). Although persons must still comply with all applicable predicate rule requirements for validation (e.g., 21 CFR 820.70(i)), this guidance should not be read to impose any additional requirements for validation.

We suggest that your decision to validate computerized systems, and the extent of the validation, take into account the impact the systems have on your ability to meet predicate rule requirements. You should also consider the impact those systems might have on the accuracy, reliability, integrity, availability, and authenticity of required records and signatures. Even if there is no predicate rule requirement to validate a system, in some instances it may still be important to validate the system.

We recommend that you base your approach on a justified and documented risk assessment and a determination of the potential of the system to affect product quality and safety, and record integrity. For instance, validation would not be important for a word processor used only to generate SOPs.

For further guidance on validation of computerized systems, see FDA's guidance for industry and FDA staff *General Principles of Software Validation* and also industry guidance such as the *GAMP 4 Guide* (See References).

2. Audit Trail

The Agency intends to exercise enforcement discretion regarding specific part 11 requirements related to computer-generated, time-stamped audit trails (§11.10 (e), (k)(2) and any corresponding requirement in §11.30). Persons must still comply with all applicable predicate rule requirements related to documentation of, for example, date (e.g., § 58.130(e)), time, or sequencing of events, as well as any requirements for ensuring that changes to records do not obscure previous entries.

Even if there are no predicate rule requirements to document, for example, date, time, or sequence of events in a particular instance, it may nonetheless be important to have audit trails or other physical, logical, or procedural security measures in place to ensure the trustworthiness and reliability of the records. [6]We recommend that you base your decision on whether to apply audit trails, or other appropriate measures, on the need to comply with predicate rule requirements, a justified and documented risk assessment, and a determination of the potential effect on product quality and safety and record integrity. We suggest that you apply appropriate controls based on such an assessment. Audit trails can be particularly appropriate when users are expected to create, modify, or delete regulated records during normal operation.

3. Legacy Systems[7]

The Agency intends to exercise enforcement discretion with respect to all part 11 requirements for systems that otherwise were operational prior to August 20, 1997, the effective date of part 11, under the circumstances specified below.

This means that the Agency does not intend to take enforcement action to enforce compliance with any part 11 requirements if all the following criteria are met for a specific system:

• The system was operational before the effective date.

• The system met all applicable predicate rule requirments before the effective date.

• The system currently meets all applicable predicate rule requirements.

• You have documented evidence and justification that the system is fit for its intended use (including having an acceptable level of record security and integrity, if applicable).

If a system has been changed since August 20, 1997, and if the changes would prevent the system from meeting predicate rule requirements, Part 11 controls should be applied to Part 11 records and signatures pursuant to the enforcement policy expressed in this guidance.

4. Copies of Records

The Agency intends to exercise enforcement discretion with regard to specific part 11 requirements for generating copies of records (§11.10 (b) and any corresponding requirement in §11.30). You should provide an investigator with reasonable and useful access to records during an inspection. All records held by you are subject to inspection in accordance with predicate rules (e.g.,§§ 211.180(c), (d), and 108.35(c)(3)(ii)).

We recommend that you supply copies of electronic records by:

• Producing copies of records held in common portable formats when records are maintained in these formats

• Using established automated conversion or export methods, where available, to make copies in a more common format (examples of such formats include, but are not limited to, PDF, XML, or SGML)

In each case, we recommend that the copying process used produces copies that preserve the content and meaning of the record. If you have the ability to search, sort, or trend part 11 records, copies given to the Agency should provide the same capability if it is reasonable and technically feasible. You should allow inspection, review, and copying of records in a human readable form at your site using your hardware and following your established procedures and techniques for accessing records.

5. Record Retention

The Agency intends to exercise enforcement discretion with regard to the part 11 requirements for the protection of records to enable their accurate and ready retrieval throughout the records retention period (§11.10 (c) and any corresponding requirement in §11.30). Persons must still comply with all applicable predicate rule requirements for record retention and availability (e.g., §§ 211.180(c),(d), 108.25(g), and 108.35(h)).

We suggest that your decision on how to maintain records be based on predicate rule requirements and that you base your decision on a justified and documented risk assessment and a determination of the value of the records over time.

FDA does not intend to object if you decide to archive required records in electronic format to nonelectronic media such as microfilm, microfiche, and paper, or to a standard electronic file format (examples of such formats include, but are not limited to, PDF, XML, or SGML). Persons must still comply with all predicate rule requirements, and the records themselves and any copies of the required records should preserve their content and meaning. As long as predicate rule requirements are fully satisfied and the content and meaning of the records are preserved and archived, you can delete the electronic version of the records. In addition, paper and electronic record and signature components can co-exist (i.e., a hybrid[8] situation) as long as predicate rule requirements are met and the content and meaning of those records are preserved.

IV. REFERENCES

Food and Drug Administration References

1. *Glossary of Computerized System and Software Development Terminology* (Division of Field Investigations, Office of Regional Operations, Office of Regulatory Affairs, FDA 1995) (http://www.fda.gov/ora/inspect_ref/igs/gloss.html)

2. *General Principles of Software Validation*; Final Guidance for Industry and FDA Staff (FDA, Center for Devices and Radiological Health, Center for Biologics Evaluation and Research, 2002) (http://www.fda.gov/cdrh/comp/guidance/938.html)

3. *Guidance for Industry, FDA Reviewers, and Compliance on Off-The-Shelf Software Use in Medical Devices* (FDA, Center for Devices and Radiological Health, 1999) (http://www.fda.gov/cdrh/ode/guidance/585.html)

4. *Pharmaceutical CGMPs for the 21st Century: A Risk-Based Approach*; A Science and Risk-Based Approach to Product Quality Regulation Incorporating an Integrated Quality Systems Approach (FDA 2002) (http://www.fda.gov/oc/guidance/gmp.html)

Industry References

1. *The Good Automated Manufacturing Practice (GAMP) Guide for Validation of Automated Systems, GAMP 4 (ISPE/GAMP Forum, 2001) (http://www.ispe.org/gamp/)*

2. ISO/IEC 17799:2000 (BS 7799:2000) Information technology - Code of practice for information security management (ISO/IEC, 2000)

3. ISO 14971:2002 Medical Devices- Application of risk management to medical devices (ISO, 2001)

[1] This guidance has been prepared by the Office of Compliance in the Center for Drug Evaluation and Research (CDER) in consultation with the other Agency centers and the Office of Regulatory Affairs at the Food and Drug Administration.

[2] 62 FR 13430

[3] These requirements include, for example, certain provisions of the Current Good Manufacturing Practice regulations (21 CFR Part 211), the Quality System regulation (21 CFR Part 820), and the Good Laboratory Practice for Nonclinical Laboratory Studies regulations (21 CFR Part 58).

[4] See Pharmaceutical CGMPs for the 21st Century: A Risk-Based Approach; A Science and Risk-Based Approach to Product Quality Regulation Incorporating an Integrated Quality Systems Approach at www.fda.gov/oc/guidance/gmp.html.

[5] Although we withdrew the draft guidance on time stamps, our current thinking has not changed in that when using time stamps for systems that span different time zones, we do not expect you to record the signer's local time. When using time stamps, they should be implemented with a clear understanding of the time zone reference used. In such instances, system documentation should explain time zone references as well as zone acronyms or other naming conventions.

[6] Various guidance documents on information security are available (see References).

[7] In this guidance document, we use the term legacy system to describe systems already in operation before the effective date of part 11.

[8] Examples of hybrid situations include combinations of paper records (or other nonelectronic media) and electronic records, paper records and electronic signatures, or handwritten signatures executed to electronic records.

Notes

Part 58

The Code of Federal Regulations
Title 21 – Food and Drugs

Part 58
GOOD LABORATORY PRACTICE
FOR NON CLINICAL
LABORATORY STUDIES

Printed by GMP Publications, Inc.
Tel: 866-544-9007 or 856-810-7331
Fax: 866-544-9002
http://www.gmppublications.com
sales@gmppublications.com

PART 58 -- GOOD LABORATORY PRACTICE FOR NONCLINICAL LABORATORY STUDIES

Subpart A -- General Provisions

Subpart B -- Organization and Personnel

Subpart C -- Facilities

Subpart D -- Equipment

Subpart E -- Testing Facilities Operation

Subpart F -- Test and Control Articles

Subpart G -- Protocol for and Conduct of a Nonclinical Laboratory Study

Subparts H-I [Reserved]

Subpart J -- Records and Reports

Subpart K -- Disqualification of Testing Facilities

Authority: 21 U.S.C. 342, 346, 346a, 348, 351, 352, 353, 355, 360, 360b-360f, 360h-360j, 371, 379e, 381; 42 U.S.C. 216, 262, 263b-263n.

Source: 43 FR 60013, Dec. 22, 1978, unless otherwise noted.

Subpart A -- General Provisions

§58.1 Scope.

(a) This part prescribes good laboratory practices for conducting nonclinical laboratory studies that support or are intended to support applications for research or marketing permits for products regulated by the Food and Drug Administration, including food and color additives, animal food additives, human and animal drugs, medical devices for human use, biological products, and electronic products. Compliance with this part is intended to assure the quality and integrity of the safety data filed pursuant to sections 406, 408, 409, 502, 503, 505, 506, 510, 512-516, 518-520, 721, and 801 of the Federal Food, Drug, and Cosmetic Act and sections 351 and 354-360F of the Public Health Service Act.

(b) References in this part to regulatory sections of the Code of Federal Regulations are to chapter I of title 21, unless otherwise noted.

[43 FR 60013, Dec. 22, 1978, as amended at 52 FR 33779, Sept. 4, 1987; 64 FR 399, Jan. 5, 1999]

§58.3 Definitions.

As used in this part, the following terms shall have the meanings specified:

(a) *Act* means the Federal Food, Drug, and Cosmetic Act, as amended (secs. 201-902, 52 Stat. 1040 et seq., as amended (21 U.S.C. 321-392)).

(b) *Test article* means any food additive, color additive, drug, biological product, electronic product, medical device for human use, or any other article subject to regulation under the act or under sections 351 and 354-360F of the Public Health Service Act.

(c) *Control article* means any food additive, color additive, drug, biological product, electronic product, medical device for human use, or any article other than a test article, feed, or water that is administered to the test system in the course of a nonclinical laboratory study for the purpose of establishing a basis for comparison with the test article.

(d) *Nonclinical laboratory study* means in vivo or in vitro experiments in which test articles are studied prospectively in test systems under laboratory conditions to determine their safety. The term does not include studies utilizing human subjects or clinical studies or field trials in animals. The term does not include basic exploratory studies carried out to determine whether a test article has any potential utility or to determine physical or chemical characteristics of a test article.

(e) *Application for research or marketing permit* includes:

(1) A color additive petition, described in part 71.

(2) A food additive petition, described in parts 171 and 571.

(3) Data and information regarding a substance submitted as part of the procedures for establishing that a substance is generally recognized as safe for use, which use results or may reasonably be expected to result, directly or indirectly, in its becoming a component or otherwise affecting the characteristics of any food, described in §§170.35 and 570.35.

(4) Data and information regarding a food additive submitted as part of the procedures regarding food additives permitted to be used on an interim basis pending additional study, described in §180.1.

(5) An *investigational new drug application*, described in part 312 of this chapter.

(6) A *new drug application*, described in part 314.

(7) Data and information regarding an over-the-counter drug for human use, submitted as part of the procedures for classifying such drugs as generally recognized as safe and effective and not misbranded, described in part 330.

(8) Data and information about a substance submitted as part of the procedures for establishing a tolerance for unavoidable contaminants in food and food-packaging materials, described in parts 109 and 509.

(9) [Reserved].

(10) A *Notice of Claimed Investigational Exemption for a New Animal Drug*, described in part 511.

(11) *A new animal drug application*, described in part 514.

(12) [Reserved]

(13) An *application for a biologics license*, described in part 601 of this chapter.

(14) An *application for an investigational device exemption*, described in part 812.

(15) An *Application for Premarket Approval of a Medical Device*, described in section 515 of the act.

(16) A *Product Development Protocol for a Medical Device*, described in section 515 of the act.

(17) Data and information regarding a medical device submitted as part of the procedures for classifying such devices, described in part 860.

(18) Data and information regarding a medical device submitted as part of the procedures for establishing, amending, or repealing a performance standard for such devices, described in part 861.

(19) Data and information regarding an electronic product submitted as part of the procedures for obtaining an exemption from notification of a radiation safety defect or failure of compliance with a radiation safety performance standard, described in subpart D of part 1003.

(20) Data and information regarding an electronic product submitted as part of the procedures for establishing, amending, or repealing a standard for such product, described in section 358 of the Public Health Service Act.

(21) Data and information regarding an electronic product submitted as part of the procedures for obtaining a variance from any electronic product performance standard as described in §1010.4.

(22) Data and information regarding an electronic product submitted as part of the procedures for granting, amending, or extending an exemption from any electronic product performance standard, as described in §1010.5.

(23) A premarket notification for a food contact substance, described in part 170, subpart D, of this chapter.

(f) *Sponsor* means:

(1) A person who initiates and supports, by provision of financial or other resources, a nonclinical laboratory study;

(2) A person who submits a nonclinical study to the Food and Drug Administration in support of an application for a research or marketing permit; or

(3) A testing facility, if it both initiates and actually conducts the study.

(g) *Testing facility* means a person who actually conducts a nonclinical laboratory study, i.e., actually uses the test article in a test system. *Testing facility* includes any establishment required to register under section 510 of the act that conducts nonclinical laboratory studies and any consulting laboratory described in section 704 of the act that conducts such studies. *Testing facility* encompasses only those operational units that are being or have been used to conduct nonclinical laboratory studies.

(h) *Person* includes an individual, partnership, corporation, association, scientific or academic establishment, government agency, or organizational unit thereof, and any other legal entity.

(i) *Test system* means any animal, plant, microorganism, or subparts thereof to which the test or control article is administered or added for study. *Test system* also includes appropriate groups or components of the system not treated with the test or control articles.

(j) *Specimen* means any material derived from a test system for examination or analysis.

(k) *Raw data* means any laboratory worksheets, records, memoranda, notes, or exact copies thereof, that are the result of original observations and activities of a nonclinical laboratory study and are necessary for the reconstruction and evaluation of the report of that study. In the event that exact transcripts of raw data have been prepared (e.g., tapes which have been transcribed verbatim, dated, and verified accurate by signature), the exact copy or exact transcript may be substituted for the original source as raw data. *Raw data* may include photographs, microfilm or microfiche copies, computer printouts, magnetic media, including dictated observations, and recorded data from automated instruments.

(l) *Quality assurance unit* means any person or organizational element, except the study director, designated by testing facility management to perform the duties relating to quality assurance of nonclinical laboratory studies.

(m) Study director means the individual responsible for the overall conduct of a nonclinical laboratory study.

(n) Batch means a specific quantity or lot of a test or control article that has been characterized according to §58.105(a).

(o) *Study initiation date* means the date the protocol is signed by the study director.

(p) *Study completion date* means the date the final report is signed by the study director.

[43 FR 60013, Dec. 22, 1978, as amended at 52 FR 33779, Sept. 4, 1987; 54 FR 9039, Mar. 3, 1989; 64 FR 56448, Oct. 20, 1999; 67 FR 35729, May 21, 2002]

§58.10   Applicability to studies performed under grants and contracts.

When a sponsor conducting a nonclinical laboratory study intended to be submitted to or reviewed by the Food and Drug Administration utilizes the services of a consulting laboratory, contractor, or grantee to perform an analysis or other service, it shall notify the consulting laboratory, contractor, or grantee that the service is part of a nonclinical laboratory study that must be conducted in compliance with the provisions of this part.

§58.15   Inspection of a testing facility.

(a) A testing facility shall permit an authorized employee of the Food and Drug Administration, at reasonable times and in a reasonable manner, to inspect the facility and to inspect (and in the case of records also to copy) all records and specimens required to be maintained regarding studies within the scope of this part. The records inspection and copying requirements shall not apply to quality assurance unit records of findings and problems, or to actions recommended and taken.

(b) The Food and Drug Administration will not consider a nonclinical laboratory study in support of an application for a research or marketing permit if the testing facility refuses to permit inspection. The determination that a nonclinical laboratory study will not be considered in support of an application for a research or marketing permit does not, however, relieve the applicant for such a permit of any obligation under any applicable statute or regulation to submit the results of the study to the Food and Drug Administration.

NOTES

Subpart B -- Organization and Personnel

§58.29   Personnel.

(a) Each individual engaged in the conduct of or responsible for the supervision of a nonclinical laboratory study shall have education, training, and experience, or combination thereof, to enable that individual to perform the assigned functions.

(b) Each testing facility shall maintain a current summary of training and experience and job description for each individual engaged in or supervising the conduct of a nonclinical laboratory study.

(c) There shall be a sufficient number of personnel for the timely and proper conduct of the study according to the protocol.

(d) Personnel shall take necessary personal sanitation and health precautions designed to avoid contamination of test and control articles and test systems.

(e) Personnel engaged in a nonclinical laboratory study shall wear clothing appropriate for the duties they perform. Such clothing shall be changed as often as necessary to prevent microbiological, radiological, or chemical contamination of test systems and test and control articles.

(f) Any individual found at any time to have an illness that may adversely affect the quality and integrity of the nonclinical laboratory study shall be excluded from direct contact with test systems, test and control articles and any other operation or function that may adversely affect the study until the condition is corrected. All personnel shall be instructed to report to their immediate supervisors any health or medical conditions that may reasonably be considered to have an adverse effect on a nonclinical laboratory study.

§58.31   Testing facility management.

For each nonclinical laboratory study, testing facility management shall:

(a) Designate a study director as described in §58.33, before the study is initiated.

(b) Replace the study director promptly if it becomes necessary to do so during the conduct of a study.

(c) Assure that there is a quality assurance unit as described in §58.35.

(d) Assure that test and control articles or mixtures have been appropriately tested for identity, strength, purity, stability, and uniformity, as applicable.

(e) Assure that personnel, resources, facilities, equipment, materials, and methodologies are available as scheduled.

(f) Assure that personnel clearly understand the functions they are to perform.

(g) Assure that any deviations from these regulations reported by the quality assurance unit are communicated to the study director and corrective actions are taken and documented.

[43 FR 60013, Dec. 22, 1978, as amended at 52 FR 33780, Sept. 4, 1987]

§58.33 Study director.

For each nonclinical laboratory study, a scientist or other professional of appropriate education, training, and experience, or combination thereof, shall be identified as the study director. The study director has overall responsibility for the technical conduct of the study, as well as for the interpretation, analysis, documentation and reporting of results, and represents the single point of study control. The study director shall assure that:

(a) The protocol, including any change, is approved as provided by §58.120 and is followed.

(b) All experimental data, including observations of unanticipated responses of the test system are accurately recorded and verified.

(c) Unforeseen circumstances that may affect the quality and integrity of the nonclinical laboratory study are noted when they occur, and corrective action is taken and documented.

(d) Test systems are as specified in the protocol.

(e) All applicable good laboratory practice regulations are followed.

(f) All raw data, documentation, protocols, specimens, and final reports are transferred to the archives during or at the close of the study.

[43 FR 60013, Dec. 22, 1978; 44 FR 17657, Mar. 23, 1979]

§58.35   Quality assurance unit.

(a) A testing facility shall have a quality assurance unit which shall be responsible for monitoring each study to assure management that the facilities, equipment, personnel, methods, practices, records, and controls are in conformance with the regulations in this part. For any given study, the quality assurance unit shall be entirely separate from and independent of the personnel engaged in the direction and conduct of that study.

(b) The quality assurance unit shall:

(1) Maintain a copy of a master schedule sheet of all nonclinical laboratory studies conducted at the testing facility indexed by test article and containing the test system, nature of study, date study was initiated, current status of each study, identity of the sponsor, and name of the study director.

(2) Maintain copies of all protocols pertaining to all nonclinical laboratory studies for which the unit is responsible.

(3) Inspect each nonclinical laboratory study at intervals adequate to assure the integrity of the study and maintain written and properly signed records of each periodic inspection showing the date of the inspection, the study inspected, the phase or segment of the study inspected, the person performing the inspection, findings and problems, action recommended and taken to resolve existing problems, and any scheduled date for reinspection. Any problems found during the course of an inspection which are likely to affect study integrity shall be brought to the attention of the study director and management immediately.

(4) Periodically submit to management and the study director written status reports on each study, noting any problems and the corrective actions taken.

(5) Determine that no deviations from approved protocols or standard operating procedures were made without proper authorization and documentation.

(6) Review the final study report to assure that such report accurately describes the methods and standard operating procedures, and that the reported results accurately reflect the raw data of the nonclinical laboratory study.

(7) Prepare and sign a statement to be included with the final study report which shall specify the dates inspections were made and findings reported to management and to the study director.

(c) The responsibilities and procedures applicable to the quality assurance unit, the records maintained by the quality assurance unit, and the method of indexing such records shall be in writing and shall be maintained. These items including inspection dates, the study inspected, the phase or segment of the study inspected, and the name of the individual performing the inspection shall be made available for inspection to authorized employees of the Food and Drug Administration.

(d) A designated representative of the Food and Drug Administration shall have access to the written procedures established for the inspection and may request testing facility management to certify that inspections are being implemented, performed, documented, and followed-up in accordance with this paragraph.

[43 FR 60013, Dec. 22, 1978, as amended at 52 FR 33780, Sept. 4, 1987; 67 FR 9585, Mar. 4, 2002]

Subpart C -- Facilities

§58.41   General.

Each testing facility shall be of suitable size and construction to facilitate the proper conduct of nonclinical laboratory studies. It shall be designed so that there is a degree of separation that will prevent any function or activity from having an adverse effect on the study.

[52 FR 33780, Sept. 4, 1987]

§58.43   Animal care facilities.

(a) A testing facility shall have a sufficient number of animal rooms or areas, as needed, to assure proper: (1) Separation of species or test systems, (2) isolation of individual projects, (3) quarantine of animals, and (4) routine or specialized housing of animals.

(b) A testing facility shall have a number of animal rooms or areas separate from those described in paragraph (a) of this section to ensure isolation of studies being done with test systems or test and control articles known to be biohazardous, including volatile substances, aerosols, radioactive materials, and infectious agents.

(c) Separate areas shall be provided, as appropriate, for the diagnosis, treatment, and control of laboratory animal diseases. These areas shall provide effective isolation for the housing of animals either known or suspected of being diseased, or of being carriers of disease, from other animals.

(d) When animals are housed, facilities shall exist for the collection and disposal of all animal waste and refuse or for safe sanitary storage of waste before removal from the testing facility. Disposal facilities shall be so provided and operated as to minimize vermin infestation, odors, disease hazards, and environmental contamination.

[43 FR 60013, Dec. 22, 1978, as amended at 52 FR 33780, Sept. 4, 1987]

§58.45   Animal supply facilities.

There shall be storage areas, as needed, for feed, bedding, supplies, and equipment. Storage areas for feed and bedding shall be separated from areas housing the test systems and shall be protected against infestation or contamination. Perishable supplies shall be preserved by appropriate means.

[43 FR 60013, Dec. 22, 1978, as amended at 52 FR 33780, Sept. 4, 1987]

§58.47   Facilities for handling test and control articles.

(a) As necessary to prevent contamination or mixups, there shall be separate areas for:

(1) Receipt and storage of the test and control articles.

(2) Mixing of the test and control articles with a carrier, e.g., feed.

(3) Storage of the test and control article mixtures.

(b) Storage areas for the test and/or control article and test and control mixtures shall be separate from areas housing the test systems and shall be adequate to preserve the identity, strength, purity, and stability of the articles and mixtures.

§58.49   Laboratory operation areas.

Separate laboratory space shall be provided, as needed, for the performance of the routine and specialized procedures required by nonclinical laboratory studies.

[52 FR 33780, Sept. 4, 1987]

§58.51   Specimen and data storage facilities.

Space shall be provided for archives, limited to access by authorized personnel only, for the storage and retrieval of all raw data and specimens from completed studies.

Subpart D -- Equipment

§58.61   Equipment design.

Equipment used in the generation, measurement, or assessment of data and equipment used for facility environmental control shall be of appropriate design and adequate capacity to function according to the protocol and shall be suitably located for operation, inspection, cleaning, and maintenance.

[52 FR 33780, Sept. 4, 1987]

§58.63   Maintenance and calibration of equipment.

(a) Equipment shall be adequately inspected, cleaned, and maintained. Equipment used for the generation, measurement, or assessment of data shall be adequately tested, calibrated and/or standardized.

(b) The written standard operating procedures required under §58.81(b)(11) shall set forth in sufficient detail the methods, materials, and schedules to be used in the routine inspection, cleaning, maintenance, testing, calibration, and/or standardization of equipment, and shall specify, when appropriate, remedial action to be taken in the event of failure or malfunction of equipment. The written standard operating procedures shall designate the person responsible for the performance of each operation.

(c) Written records shall be maintained of all inspection, maintenance, testing, calibrating and/or standardizing operations. These records, containing the date of the operation, shall describe whether the maintenance operations were routine and followed the written standard operating procedures. Written records shall be kept of nonroutine repairs performed on equipment as a result of failure and malfunction. Such records shall document the nature of the defect, how and when the defect was discovered, and any remedial action taken in response to the defect.

[43 FR 60013, Dec. 22, 1978, as amended at 52 FR 33780, Sept. 4, 1987; 67 FR 9585, Mar. 4, 2002]

Subpart E -- Testing Facilities Operation

§58.81 Standard operating procedures.

(a) A testing facility shall have standard operating procedures in writing setting forth nonclinical laboratory study methods that management is satisfied are adequate to insure the quality and integrity of the data generated in the course of a study. All deviations in a study from standard operating procedures shall be authorized by the study director and shall be documented in the raw data. Significant changes in established standard operating procedures shall be properly authorized in writing by management.

(b) Standard operating procedures shall be established for, but not limited to, the following:

(1) Animal room preparation.

(2) Animal care.

(3) Receipt, identification, storage, handling, mixing, and method of sampling of the test and control articles.

(4) Test system observations.

(5) Laboratory tests.

(6) Handling of animals found moribund or dead during study.

(7) Necropsy of animals or postmortem examination of animals.

(8) Collection and identification of specimens.

(9) Histopathology.

(10) Data handling, storage, and retrieval.

(11) Maintenance and calibration of equipment.

(12) Transfer, proper placement, and identification of animals.

(c) Each laboratory area shall have immediately available laboratory manuals and standard operating procedures relative to the laboratory procedures being performed. Published literature may be used as a supplement to standard operating procedures.

(d) A historical file of standard operating procedures, and all revisions thereof, including the dates of such revisions, shall be maintained.

[43 FR 60013, Dec. 22, 1978, as amended at 52 FR 33780, Sept. 4, 1987]

§58.83   Reagents and solutions.

All reagents and solutions in the laboratory areas shall be labeled to indicate identity, titer or concentration, storage requirements, and expiration date. Deteriorated or outdated reagents and solutions shall not be used.

§58.90   Animal care.

(a) There shall be standard operating procedures for the housing, feeding, handling, and care of animals.

(b) All newly received animals from outside sources shall be isolated and their health status shall be evaluated in accordance with acceptable veterinary medical practice.

(c) At the initiation of a nonclinical laboratory study, animals shall be free of any disease or condition that might interfere with the purpose or conduct of the study. If, during the course of the study, the animals contract such a disease or condition, the diseased animals shall be isolated, if necessary. These animals may be treated for disease or signs of disease provided that such treatment does not interfere with the study. The diagnosis, authorizations of treatment, description of treatment, and each date of treatment shall be documented and shall be retained.

(d) Warm-blooded animals, excluding suckling rodents, used in laboratory procedures that require manipulations and observations over an extended period of time or in studies that require the animals to be removed from and returned to their home cages for any reason (e.g., cage cleaning, treatment, etc.), shall receive appropriate identification. All information needed to specifically identify each animal within an animal-housing unit shall appear on the outside of that unit.

(e) Animals of different species shall be housed in separate rooms when necessary. Animals of the same species, but used in different studies, should not ordinarily be housed in the same room when inadvertent exposure to control or test articles or animal mixup could affect the outcome of either study. If such mixed housing is necessary, adequate differentiation by space and identification shall be made.

(f) Animal cages, racks and accessory equipment shall be cleaned and sanitized at appropriate intervals.

(g) Feed and water used for the animals shall be analyzed periodically to ensure that contaminants known to be capable of interfering with the study and reasonably expected to be present in such feed or water are not present at levels above those specified in the protocol. Documentation of such analyses shall be maintained as raw data.

(h) Bedding used in animal cages or pens shall not interfere with the purpose or conduct of the study and shall be changed as often as necessary to keep the animals dry and clean.

(i) If any pest control materials are used, the use shall be documented. Cleaning and pest control materials that interfere with the study shall not be used.

[43 FR 60013, Dec. 22, 1978, as amended at 52 FR 33780, Sept. 4, 1987; 54 FR 15924, Apr. 20, 1989; 56 FR 32088, July 15, 1991; 67 FR 9585, Mar. 4, 2002]

NOTES

Subpart F -- Test and Control Articles

§58.105 Test and control article characterization.

(a) The identity, strength, purity, and composition or other characteristics which will appropriately define the test or control article shall be determined for each batch and shall be documented. Methods of synthesis, fabrication, or derivation of the test and control articles shall be documented by the sponsor or the testing facility. In those cases where marketed products are used as control articles, such products will be characterized by their labeling.

(b) The stability of each test or control article shall be determined by the testing facility or by the sponsor either: (1) Before study initiation, or (2) concomitantly according to written standard operating procedures, which provide for periodic analysis of each batch.

(c) Each storage container for a test or control article shall be labeled by name, chemical abstract number or code number, batch number, expiration date, if any, and, where appropriate, storage conditions necessary to maintain the identity, strength, purity, and composition of the test or control article. Storage containers shall be assigned to a particular test article for the duration of the study.

(d) For studies of more than 4 weeks' duration, reserve samples from each batch of test and control articles shall be retained for the period of time provided by §58.195.

[43 FR 60013, Dec. 22, 1978, as amended at 52 FR 33781, Sept. 4, 1987; 67 FR 9585, Mar. 4, 2002]

§58.107 Test and control article handling.

Procedures shall be established for a system for the handling of the test and control articles to ensure that:

(a) There is proper storage.

(b) Distribution is made in a manner designed to preclude the possibility of contamination, deterioration, or damage.

(c) Proper identification is maintained throughout the distribution process.

(d) The receipt and distribution of each batch is documented. Such documentation shall include the date and quantity of each batch distributed or returned.

§58.113   Mixtures of articles with carriers.

(a) For each test or control article that is mixed with a carrier, tests by appropriate analytical methods shall be conducted:

(1) To determine the uniformity of the mixture and to determine, periodically, the concentration of the test or control article in the mixture.

(2) To determine the stability of the test and control articles in the mixture as required by the conditions of the study either:

(i) Before study initiation, or

(ii) Concomitantly according to written standard operating procedures which provide for periodic analysis of the test and control articles in the mixture.

(b) [Reserved]

(c) Where any of the components of the test or control article carrier mixture has an expiration date, that date shall be clearly shown on the container. If more than one component has an expiration date, the earliest date shall be shown.

[43 FR 60013, Dec. 22, 1978, as amended at 45 FR 24865, Apr. 11, 1980; 52 FR 33781, Sept. 4, 1987]

Subpart G -- Protocol for and Conduct of a Nonclinical Laboratory Study

§58.120   Protocol.

(a) Each study shall have an approved written protocol that clearly indicates the objectives and all methods for the conduct of the study. The protocol shall contain, as applicable, the following information:

(1) A descriptive title and statement of the purpose of the study.

(2) Identification of the test and control articles by name, chemical abstract number, or code number.

(3) The name of the sponsor and the name and address of the testing facility at which the study is being conducted.

(4) The number, body weight range, sex, source of supply, species, strain, substrain, and age of the test system.

(5) The procedure for identification of the test system.

(6) A description of the experimental design, including the methods for the control of bias.

(7) A description and/or identification of the diet used in the study as well as solvents, emulsifiers, and/or other materials used to solubilize or suspend the test or control articles before mixing with the carrier. The description shall include specifications for acceptable levels of contaminants that are reasonably expected to be present in the dietary materials and are known to be capable of interfering with the purpose or conduct of the study if present at levels greater than established by the specifications.

(8) Each dosage level, expressed in milligrams per kilogram of body weight or other appropriate units, of the test or control article to be administered and the method and frequency of administration.

(9) The type and frequency of tests, analyses, and measurements to be made.

(10) The records to be maintained.

(11) The date of approval of the protocol by the sponsor and the dated signature of the study director.

(12) A statement of the proposed statistical methods to be used.

(b) All changes in or revisions of an approved protocol and the reasons therefor shall be documented, signed by the study director, dated, and maintained with the protocol.

[43 FR 60013, Dec. 22, 1978, as amended at 52 FR 33781, Sept. 4, 1987; 67 FR 9585, Mar. 4, 2002]

§58.130 Conduct of a nonclinical laboratory study.

(a) The nonclinical laboratory study shall be conducted in accordance with the protocol.

(b) The test systems shall be monitored in conformity with the protocol.

(c) Specimens shall be identified by test system, study, nature, and date of collection. This information shall be located on the specimen container or shall accompany the specimen in a manner that precludes error in the recording and storage of data.

(d) Records of gross findings for a specimen from post-mortem observations should be available to a pathologist when examining that specimen histopathologically.

(e) All data generated during the conduct of a nonclinical laboratory study, except those that are generated by automated data collection systems, shall be recorded directly, promptly, and legibly in ink. All data entries shall be dated on the date of entry and signed or initialed by the person entering the data. Any change in entries shall be made so as not to obscure the original entry, shall indicate the reason for such change, and shall be dated and signed or identified at the time of the change. In automated data collection systems, the individual responsible for direct data input shall be identified at the time of data input. Any change in automated data entries shall be made so as not to obscure the original entry, shall indicate the reason for change, shall be dated, and the responsible individual shall be identified.

[43 FR 60013, Dec. 22, 1978, as amended at 52 FR 33781, Sept. 4, 1987; 67 FR 9585, Mar. 4, 2002]

Subparts H-I [Reserved]

Subpart J -- Records and Reports

§58.185   Reporting of nonclinical laboratory study results.

(a) A final report shall be prepared for each nonclinical laboratory study and shall include, but not necessarily be limited to, the following:

(1) Name and address of the facility performing the study and the dates on which the study was initiated and completed.

(2) Objectives and procedures stated in the approved protocol, including any changes in the original protocol.

(3) Statistical methods employed for analyzing the data.

(4) The test and control articles identified by name, chemical abstracts number or code number, strength, purity, and composition or other appropriate characteristics.

(5) Stability of the test and control articles under the conditions of administration.

(6) A description of the methods used.

(7) A description of the test system used. Where applicable, the final report shall include the number of animals used, sex, body weight range, source of supply, species, strain and substrain, age, and procedure used for identification.

(8) A description of the dosage, dosage regimen, route of administration, and duration.

(9) A description of all cirmcumstances that may have affected the quality or integrity of the data.

(10) The name of the study director, the names of other scientists or professionals, and the names of all supervisory personnel, involved in the study.

(11) A description of the transformations, calculations, or operations performed on the data, a summary and analysis of the data, and a statement of the conclusions drawn from the analysis.

(12) The signed and dated reports of each of the individual scientists or other professionals involved in the study.

(13) The locations where all specimens, raw data, and the final report are to be stored.

(14) The statement prepared and signed by the quality assurance unit as described in §58.35(b)(7).

(b) The final report shall be signed and dated by the study director.

(c) Corrections or additions to a final report shall be in the form of an amendment by the study director. The amendment shall clearly identify that part of the final report that is being added to or corrected and the reasons for the correction or addition, and shall be signed and dated by the person responsible.

[43 FR 60013, Dec. 22, 1978, as amended at 52 FR 33781, Sept. 4, 1987]

§58.190   Storage and retrieval of records and data.

(a) All raw data, documentation, protocols, final reports, and specimens (except those specimens obtained from mutagenicity tests and wet specimens of blood, urine, feces, and biological fluids) generated as a result of a nonclinical laboratory study shall be retained.

(b) There shall be archives for orderly storage and expedient retrieval of all raw data, documentation, protocols, specimens, and interim and final reports. Conditions of storage shall minimize deterioration of the documents or specimens in accordance with the requirements for the time period of their retention and the nature of the documents or specimens. A testing facility may contract with commercial archives to provide a repository for all material to be retained. Raw data and specimens may be retained elsewhere provided that the archives have specific reference to those other locations.

(c) An individual shall be identified as responsible for the archives.

(d) Only authorized personnel shall enter the archives.

(e) Material retained or referred to in the archives shall be indexed to permit expedient retrieval.

[43 FR 60013, Dec. 22, 1978, as amended at 52 FR 33781, Sept. 4, 1987; 67 FR 9585, Mar. 4, 2002]

§58.195   Retention of records.

(a) Record retention requirements set forth in this section do not supersede the record retention requirements of any other regulations in this chapter.

(b) Except as provided in paragraph (c) of this section, documentation records, raw data and specimens pertaining to a nonclinical laboratory study and required to be made by this part shall be retained in the archive(s) for whichever of the following periods is shortest:

(1) A period of at least 2 years following the date on which an application for a research or marketing permit, in support of which the results of the nonclinical laboratory study were submitted, is approved by the Food and Drug Administration. This requirement does not apply to studies supporting investigational new drug applications (IND's) or applications for investigational device exemptions (IDE's), records of which shall be governed by the provisions of paragraph (b)(2) of this section.

(2) A period of at least 5 years following the date on which the results of the nonclinical laboratory study are submitted to the Food and Drug Administration in support of an application for a research or marketing permit.

(3) In other situations (e.g., where the nonclinical laboratory study does not result in the submission of the study in support of an application for a research or marketing permit), a period of at least 2 years following the date on which the study is completed, terminated, or discontinued.

(c) Wet specimens (except those specimens obtained from mutagenicity tests and wet specimens of blood, urine, feces, and biological fluids), samples of test or control articles, and specially prepared material, which are relatively fragile and differ markedly in stability and quality during storage, shall be retained only as long as the quality of the preparation affords evaluation. In no case shall retention be required for longer periods than those set forth in paragraphs (a) and (b) of this section.

(d) The master schedule sheet, copies of protocols, and records of quality assurance inspections, as required by §58.35(c) shall be maintained by the quality assurance unit as an easily accessible system of records for the period of time specified in paragraphs (a) and (b) of this section.

(e) Summaries of training and experience and job descriptions required to be maintained by §58.29(b) may be retained along with all other testing facility employment records for the length of time specified in paragraphs (a) and (b) of this section.

(f) Records and reports of the maintenance and calibration and inspection of equipment, as required by §58.63(b) and (c), shall be retained for the length of time specified in paragraph (b) of this section.

(g) Records required by this part may be retained either as original records or as true copies such as photocopies, microfilm, microfiche, or other accurate reproductions of the original records.

(h) If a facility conducting nonclinical testing goes out of business, all raw data, documentation, and other material specified in this section shall be transferred to the archives of the sponsor of the study. The Food and Drug Administration shall be notified in writing of such a transfer.

[43 FR 60013, Dec. 22, 1978, as amended at 52 FR 33781, Sept. 4, 1987; 54 FR 9039, Mar. 3, 1989]

Subpart K -- Disqualification of Testing Facilities

§58.200   Purpose.

(a) The purposes of disqualification are:

(1) To permit the exclusion from consideration of completed studies that were conducted by a testing facility which has failed to comply with the requirements of the good laboratory practice regulations until it can be adequately demonstrated that such noncompliance did not occur during, or did not affect the validity or acceptability of data generated by, a particular study; and

(2) To exclude from consideration all studies completed after the date of disqualification until the facility can satisfy the Commissioner that it will conduct studies in compliance with such regulations.

(b) The determination that a nonclinical laboratory study may not be considered in support of an application for a research or marketing permit does not, however, relieve the applicant for such a permit of any obligation under any other applicable regulation to submit the results of the study to the Food and Drug Administration.

§58.202   Grounds for disqualification.

The Commissioner may disqualify a testing facility upon finding all of the following:

(a) The testing facility failed to comply with one or more of the regulations set forth in this part (or any other regulations regarding such facilities in this chapter);

(b) The noncompliance adversely affected the validity of the nonclinical laboratory studies; and

(c) Other lesser regulatory actions (e.g., warnings or rejection of individual studies) have not been or will probably not be adequate to achieve compliance with the good laboratory practice regulations.

§58.204   Notice of and opportunity for hearing on proposed disqualification.

(a) Whenever the Commissioner has information indicating that grounds exist under §58.202 which in his opinion justify disqualification of a testing facility, he may issue to the testing facility a written notice proposing that the facility be disqualified.

(b) A hearing on the disqualification shall be conducted in accordance with the requirements for a regulatory hearing set forth in part 16 of this chapter.

§58.206   Final order on disqualification.

(a) If the Commissioner, after the regulatory hearing, or after the time for requesting a hearing expires without a request being made, upon an evaluation of the administrative record of the disqualification proceeding, makes the findings required in §58.202, he shall issue a final order disqualifying the facility. Such order shall include a statement of the basis for that determination. Upon issuing a final order, the Commissioner shall notify (with a copy of the order) the testing facility of the action.

(b) If the Commissioner, after a regulatory hearing or after the time for requesting a hearing expires without a request being made, upon an evaluation of the administrative record of the disqualification proceeding, does not make the findings required in §58.202, he shall issue a final order terminating the disqualification proceeding. Such order shall include a statement of the basis for that determination. Upon issuing a final order the Commissioner shall notify the testing facility and provide a copy of the order.

§58.210   Actions upon disqualification.

(a) Once a testing facility has been disqualified, each application for a research or marketing permit, whether approved or not, containing or relying upon any nonclinical laboratory study conducted by the disqualified testing facility may be examined to determine whether such study was or would be essential to a decision. If it is determined that a study was or would be essential, the Food and Drug Administration shall also determine whether the study is acceptable, notwithstanding the disqualification of the facility. Any study done by a testing facility before or after disqualification may be presumed to be unacceptable, and the person relying on the study may be required to establish that the study was not affected by the circumstances that led to the disqualification, e.g., by submitting validating information. If the study is then determined to be unacceptable, such data will be eliminated from consideration in support of the application; and such elimination may serve as new information justifying the termination or withdrawal of approval of the application.

(b) No nonclinical laboratory study begun by a testing facility after the date of the facility's disqualification shall be considered in support of any application for a research or marketing permit, unless the facility has been reinstated under §58.219. The determination that a study may not be considered in support of an application for a research or marketing permit does not, however, relieve the applicant for such a permit of any obligation under any other applicable regulation to submit the results of the study to the Food and Drug Administration.

[43 FR 60013, Dec. 22, 1978, as amended at 59 FR 13200, Mar. 21, 1994]

§58.213   Public disclosure of information regarding disqualification.

(a) Upon issuance of a final order disqualifying a testing facility under §58.206(a), the Commissioner may notify all or any interested persons. Such notice may be given at the discretion of the Commissioner whenever he believes that such disclosure would further the public interest or would promote compliance with the good laboratory practice regulations set forth in this part. Such notice, if given, shall include a copy of the final order issued under §58.206(a) and shall state that the disqualification constitutes a determination by the Food and Drug Administration that nonclinical laboratory studies performed by the facility will not be considered by the Food and Drug Administration in support of any application for a research or marketing permit. If such notice is sent to another Federal Government agency, the Food and Drug Administration will recommend that the agency also consider whether or not it should accept nonclinical laboratory studies performed by the testing facility. If such notice is sent to any other person, it shall state that it is given because of the relationship between the testing facility and the person being notified and that the Food and Drug Administration is not advising or recommending that any action be taken by the person notified.

(b) A determination that a testing facility has been disqualified and the administrative record regarding such determination are disclosable to the public under part 20 of this chapter.

§58.215   Alternative or additional actions to disqualification.

(a) Disqualification of a testing facility under this subpart is independent of, and neither in lieu of nor a precondition to, other proceedings or actions authorized by the act. The Food and Drug Administration may, at any time, institute against a testing facility and/or against the sponsor of a nonclinical laboratory study that has been submitted to the Food and Drug Administration any appropriate judicial proceedings (civil or criminal) and any other appropriate regulatory action, in addition to or in lieu of, and prior to, simultaneously with, or subsequent to, disqualification. The Food and Drug Administration may also refer the matter to another Federal, State, or local government law enforcement or regulatory agency for such action as that agency deems appropriate.

(b) The Food and Drug Administration may refuse to consider any particular nonclinical laboratory study in support of an application for a research or marketing permit, if it finds that the study was not conducted in accordance with the good laboratory practice regulations set forth in this part, without disqualifying the testing facility that conducted the study or undertaking other regulatory action.

§58.217 Suspension or termination of a testing facility by a sponsor.

Termination of a testing facility by a sponsor is independent of, and neither in lieu of nor a precondition to, proceedings or actions authorized by this subpart. If a sponsor terminates or suspends a testing facility from further participation in a nonclinical laboratory study that is being conducted as part of any application for a research or marketing permit that has been submitted to any Center of the Food and Drug Administration (whether approved or not), it shall notify that Center in writing within 15 working days of the action; the notice shall include a statement of the reasons for such action. Suspension or termination of a testing facility by a sponsor does not relieve it of any obligation under any other applicable regulation to submit the results of the study to the Food and Drug Administration.

[43 FR FR 60013, Dec. 22, 1978, as amended at 50 FR 8995, Mar. 6, 1985]

§58.219 Reinstatement of a disqualified testing facility.

A testing facility that has been disqualified may be reinstated as an acceptable source of nonclinical laboratory studies to be submitted to the Food and Drug Administration if the Commissioner determines, upon an evaluation of the submission of the testing facility, that the facility can adequately assure that it will conduct future nonclinical laboratory studies in compliance with the good laboratory practice regulations set forth in this part and, if any studies are currently being conducted, that the quality and integrity of such studies have not been seriously compromised. A disqualified testing facility that wishes to be so reinstated shall present in writing to the Commissioner reasons why it believes it should be reinstated and a detailed description of the corrective actions it has taken or intends to take to assure that the acts or omissions which led to its disqualification will not recur. The Commissioner may condition reinstatement upon the testing facility being found in compliance with the good laboratory practice regulations upon an inspection. If a testing facility is reinstated, the Commissioner shall so notify the testing facility and all organizations and persons who were notified, under §58.213 of the disqualification of the testing facility. A determination that a testing facility has been reinstated is disclosable to the public under part 20 of this chapter.

NOTES

Notes

_____

_____

_____

_____

_____

_____

_____

_____

_____

_____

_____

_____

_____

_____

_____

_____

_____

Parts 210 & 211

The Code of Federal Regulations
Title 21 – Food and Drugs

Parts 210 & 211
cGMP in Manufacturing, Processing, Packing, or Holding of Drugs and Finished Pharmaceuticals

---

Printed by GMP Publications, Inc.
Tel: 866-544-9007 or 856-810-7331
Fax: 866-544-9002
http://www.gmppublications.com
sales@gmppublications.com

PART 210--CURRENT GOOD MANUFACTURING PRACTICE IN MANUFACTURING, PROCESSING, PACKING, OR HOLDING OF DRUGS; GENERAL

Authority: 21 U.S.C. 321, 351, 352, 355, 360b, 371, 374; 42 U.S.C. 216, 262, 263a, 264.
Source: 43 FR 45076, Sept, 29, 1978, unless otherwise noted.

§210.1   Status of current good manufacturing practice regulations.

(a) The regulations set forth in this part and in parts 211, 225, and 226 of this chapter contain the minimum current good manufacturing practice for methods to be used in, and the facilities or controls to be used for, the manufacture, processing, packing, or holding of a drug to assure that such drug meets the requirements of the act as to safety, and has the identity and strength and meets the quality and purity characteristics that it purports or is represented to possess.

(b) The failure to comply with any regulation set forth in this part and in parts 211, 225, and 226 of this chapter in the manufacture, processing, packing, or holding of a drug shall render such drug to be adulterated under section 501(a)(2)(B) of the act and such drug, as well as the person who is responsible for the failure to comply, shall be subject to regulatory action.

(c) Owners and operators of establishments engaged in the recovery, donor screening, testing (including donor testing), processing, storage, labeling, packaging, or distribution of human cells, tissues, and cellular and tissue-based products (HCT/Ps), as defined in §1271.3(d) of this chapter, that are drugs (subject to review under an application submitted under section 505 of the act or under a biological product license application under section 351 of the Public Health Service Act), are subject to the donor-eligibility and applicable current good tissue practice procedures set forth in part 1271 subparts C and D of this chapter, in addition to the regulations in this part and in parts 211, 225, and 226 of this chapter. Failure to comply with any applicable regulation set forth in this part, in parts 211, 225, and 226 of this chapter, in part 1271 subpart C of this chapter, or in part 1271 subpart D of this chapter with respect to the manufacture, processing, packing or holding of a drug, renders an HCT/P adulterated under section 501(a)(2)(B) of the act. Such HCT/P, as well as the person who is responsible for the failure to comply, is subject to regulatory action.

[43 FR 45076, Sept. 29, 1978, as amended at 69 FR 29828, May 25, 2004; 74 FR 65431, Dec. 10, 2009]

§210.2 Applicability of current good manufacturing practice regulations.

(a) The regulations in this part and in parts 211, 225, and 226 of this chapter as they may pertain to a drug; in parts 600 through 680 of this chapter as they may pertain to a biological product for human use; and in part 1271 of this chapter as they are applicable to a human cell, tissue, or cellular or tissue-based product (HCT/P) that is a drug (subject to review under an application submitted under section 505 of the act or under a biological product license application under section 351 of the Public Health Service Act); shall be considered to supplement, not supersede, each other, unless the regulations explicitly provide otherwise. In the event of a conflict between applicable regulations in this part and in other parts of this chapter, the regulation specifically applicable to the drug product in question shall supersede the more general.

(b) If a person engages in only some operations subject to the regulations in this part, in parts 211, 225, and 226 of this chapter, in parts 600 through 680 of this chapter, and in part 1271 of this chapter, and not in others, that person need only comply with those regulations applicable to the operations in which he or she is engaged.

(c) An investigational drug for use in a phase 1 study, as described in §312.21(a) of this chapter, is subject to the statutory requirements set forth in 21 U.S.C. 351(a)(2)(B). The production of such drug is exempt from compliance with the regulations in part 211 of this chapter. However, this exemption does not apply to an investigational drug for use in a phase 1 study once the investigational drug has been made available for use by or for the sponsor in a phase 2 or phase 3 study, as described in §312.21(b) and (c) of this chapter, or the drug has been lawfully marketed. If the investigational drug has been made available in a phase 2 or phase 3 study or the drug has been lawfully marketed, the drug for use in the phase 1 study must comply with part 211.

[69 FR 29828, May 25, 2004, as amended at 73 FR 40462, July 15, 2008; 74 FR 65431, Dec. 10, 2009]

§210.3 Definitions.

(a) The definitions and interpretations contained in section 201 of the act shall be applicable to such terms when used in this part and in parts 211, 225, and 226 of this chapter.

(b) The following definitions of terms apply to this part and to parts 211 through 226 of this chapter.

(1) *Act* means the Federal Food, Drug, and Cosmetic Act, as amended (21 U.S.C. 301 *et seq.*).

(2) *Batch* means a specific quantity of a drug or other material that is intended to have uniform character and quality, within specified limits, and is produced according to a single manufacturing order during the same cycle of manufacture.

(3) *Component* means any ingredient intended for use in the manufacture of a drug product, including those that may not appear in such drug product.

(4) *Drug product* means a finished dosage form, for example, tablet, capsule, solution, etc., that contains an active drug ingredient generally, but not necessarily, in association with inactive ingredients. The term also includes a finished dosage form that does not contain an active ingredient but is intended to be used as a placebo.

(5) *Fiber* means any particulate contaminant with a length at least three times greater than its width.

(6) *Nonfiber releasing filter* means any filter, which after appropriate pretreatment such as washing or flushing,

will not release fibers into the component or drug product that is being filtered.

(7) *Active ingredient* means any component that is intended to furnish pharmacological activity or other direct effect in the diagnosis, cure, mitigation, treatment, or prevention of disease, or to affect the structure or any function of the body of man or other animals. The term includes those components that may undergo chemical change in the manufacture of the drug product and be present in the drug product in a modified form intended to furnish the specified activity or effect.

(8) *Inactive ingredient* means any component other than an active ingredient.

(9) *In-process material* means any material fabricated, compounded, blended, or derived by chemical reaction that is produced for, and used in, the preparation of the drug product.

(10) *Lot* means a batch, or a specific identified portion of a batch, having uniform character and quality within specified limits; or, in the case of a drug product produced by continuous process, it is a specific identified amount produced in a unit of time or quantity in a manner that assures its having uniform character and quality within specified limits.

(11) *Lot number, control number, or batch number* means any distinctive combination of letters, numbers, or symbols, or any combination of them, from which the complete history of the manufacture, processing, packing, holding, and distribution of a batch or lot of drug product or other material can be determined.

(12) *Manufacture, processing, packing, or holding of a drug product* includes packaging and labeling operations, testing, and quality control of drug products.

(13) The term *medicated feed* means any Type B or Type C medicated feed as defined in §558.3 of this chapter. The feed contains one or more drugs as defined in section 201(g) of the act. The manufacture of medicated feeds is subject to the requirements of part 225 of this chapter.

(14) The term *medicated premix* means a Type A medicated article as defined in §558.3 of this chapter. The article contains one or more drugs as defined in section

201(g) of the act. The manufacture of medicated premixes is subject to the requirements of part 226 of this chapter.

(15) *Quality control unit* means any person or organizational element designated by the firm to be responsible for the duties relating to quality control.

(16) *Strength* means:

(i) The concentration of the drug substance (for example, weight/weight, weight/volume, or unit dose/volume basis), and/or

(ii) The potency, that is, the therapeutic activity of the drug product as indicated by appropriate laboratory tests or by adequately developed and controlled clinical data (expressed, for example, in terms of units by reference to a standard).

(17) *Theoretical yield* means the quantity that would be produced at any appropriate phase of manufacture, processing, or packing of a particular drug product, based upon the quantity of components to be used, in the absence of any loss or error in actual production.

(18) *Actual yield* means the quantity that is actually produced at any appropriate phase of manufacture, processing, or packing of a particular drug product.

(19) *Percentage of theoretical yield* means the ratio of the actual yield (at any appropriate phase of manufacture, processing, or packing of a particular drug product) to the theoretical yield (at the same phase), stated as a percentage.

(20) *Acceptance criteria* means the product specifications and acceptance/rejection criteria, such as acceptable quality level and unacceptable quality level, with an associated sampling plan, that are necessary for making a decision to accept or reject a lot or batch (or any other convenient subgroups of manufactured units).

(21) *Representative sample* means a sample that consists of a number of units that are drawn based on rational criteria such as random sampling and intended to assure that the sample accurately portrays the material being sampled.

(22) *Gang-printed labeling* means labeling derived from a sheet of material on which more than one item of labeling is printed.

[43 FR 45076, Sept. 29, 1978, as amended at 51 FR 7389, Mar. 3, 1986; 58 FR 41353, Aug. 3, 1993; 73 FR 51931, Sept. 8, 2008; 74 FR 65431, Dec. 10, 2009]

PART 211--CURRENT GOOD MANUFACTURING PRACTICE FOR FINISHED PHARMACEUTICALS

Subpart A--General Provisions

Subpart B--Organization and Personnel

Subpart C--Buildings and Facilities

Subpart D--Equipment

Subpart E--Control of Components and Drug Product Containers and Closures

Subpart J--Records and Reports

Subpart K--Returned and Salvaged Drug Products

Authority: 21 U.S.C. 321, 351, 352, 355, 360b, 371, 374; 42 U.S.C. 216, 262, 263a, 264.

Source: 43 FR 45077, Sept. 29, 1978, unless otherwise noted.

Subpart A--General Provisions

§211.1   Scope.

(a) The regulations in this part contain the minimum current good manufacturing practice for preparation of drug products (excluding positron emission tomography drugs) for administration to humans or animals.

(b) The current good manufacturing practice regulations in this chapter as they pertain to drug products; in parts 600 through 680 of this chapter, as they pertain to drugs that are also biological products for human use; and in part 1271 of this chapter, as they are applicable to drugs that are also human cells, tissues, and cellular and tissue-based products (HCT/Ps) and that are drugs (subject to review under an application submitted under section 505 of the act or under a biological product license application under section 351 of the Public Health Service Act); supplement and do not supersede the regulations in this part unless the regulations explicitly provide otherwise. In the event of a conflict between applicable regulations in this part and in other parts of this chapter, or in parts 600 through 680 of this chapter, or in part 1271 of this chapter, the regulation specifically applicable to the drug product in question shall supersede the more general.

(c) Pending consideration of a proposed exemption, published in the FEDERAL REGISTER of September 29, 1978, the requirements in this part shall not be enforced for OTC drug products if the products and all their ingredients are ordinarily marketed and consumed as human foods, and which products may also fall within the legal definition of drugs by virtue of their intended use. Therefore, until further notice, regulations under parts 110 and 117 of this chapter, and where applicable, parts 113 through 129 of this chapter, shall be applied in determining whether these OTC drug products that are also foods are manufactured, processed, packed, or held under current good manufacturing practice.

[43 FR 45077, Sept. 29, 1978, as amended at 62 FR 66522, Dec. 19, 1997; 69 FR 29828, May 25, 2004; 74 FR 65431, Dec. 10, 2009; 80 FR 56168, Sept. 17, 2015]

§211.3 Definitions.

The definitions set forth in §210.3 of this chapter apply in this part.

Subpart B--Organization and Personnel

§211.22 Responsibilities of quality control unit.

(a) There shall be a quality control unit that shall have the responsibility and authority to approve or reject all components, drug product containers, closures, in-process materials, packaging material, labeling, and drug products, and the authority to review production records to assure that no errors have occurred or, if errors have occurred, that they have been fully investigated. The quality control unit shall be responsible for approving or rejecting drug products manufactured, processed, packed, or held under contract by another company.

(b) Adequate laboratory facilities for the testing and approval (or rejection) of components, drug product containers, closures, packaging materials, in-process materials, and drug products shall be available to the quality control unit.

(c) The quality control unit shall have the responsibility for approving or rejecting all procedures or specifications impacting on the identity, strength, quality, and purity of the drug product.

(d) The responsibilities and procedures applicable to the quality control unit shall be in writing; such written procedures shall be followed.

§211.25 Personnel qualifications.

(a) Each person engaged in the manufacture, processing, packing, or holding of a drug product shall have education, training, and experience, or any combination thereof, to enable that person to perform the assigned functions. Training shall be in the particular operations that the employee performs and in current good manufacturing practice (including the current good manufacturing practice regulations in this chapter and written procedures required by these regulations) as they relate to the employee's functions. Training in current good manufacturing practice shall be conducted by qualified individuals on a continuing basis and with sufficient frequency to assure that employees remain familiar with CGMP requirements applicable to them.

(b) Each person responsible for supervising the manufacture, processing, packing, or holding of a drug product shall have the education, training, and experience, or any combination thereof, to perform assigned functions in such a manner as to provide assurance that the drug product has the safety, identity, strength, quality, and purity that it purports or is represented to possess.

(c) There shall be an adequate number of qualified personnel to perform and supervise the manufacture, processing, packing, or holding of each drug product.

§211.28   Personnel responsibilities.

(a) Personnel engaged in the manufacture, processing, packing, or holding of a drug product shall wear clean clothing appropriate for the duties they perform. Protective apparel, such as head, face, hand, and arm coverings, shall be worn as necessary to protect drug products from contamination.

(b) Personnel shall practice good sanitation and health habits.

(c) Only personnel authorized by supervisory personnel shall enter those areas of the buildings and facilities designated as limited-access areas.

d) Any person shown at any time (either by medical examination or supervisory observation) to have an apparent illness or open lesions that may adversely affect the safety or quality of drug products shall be excluded from direct contact with components, drug product containers, closures, in-process materials, and drug products until the condition is corrected or determined by competent medical personnel not to jeopardize the safety or quality of drug products. All personnel shall be instructed to report to supervisory personnel any health conditions that may have an adverse effect on drug products.

§211.34　　Consultants.

Consultants advising on the manufacture, processing, packing, or holding of drug products shall have sufficient education, training, and experience, or any combination thereof, to advise on the subject for which they are retained. Records shall be maintained stating the name, address, and qualifications of any consultants and the type of service they provide.

Subpart C--Buildings and Facilities

§211.42　　Design and construction features.

(a) Any building or buildings used in the manufacture, processing, packing, or holding of a drug product shall be of suitable size, construction and location to facilitate cleaning, maintenance, and proper operations.

(b) Any such building shall have adequate space for the orderly placement of equipment and materials to prevent mixups between different components, drug product containers, closures, labeling, in-process materials, or drug products, and to prevent contamination. The flow of components, drug product containers, closures, labeling, in-process materials, and drug products through the building or buildings shall be designed to prevent contamination.

(c) Operations shall be performed within specifically defined areas of adequate size. There shall be separate or defined areas or such other control systems for the firm's operations as are necessary to prevent contamination or mixups during the course of the following procedures:

(1) Receipt, identification, storage, and withholding from use of components, drug product containers, closures, and labeling, pending the appropriate sampling, testing, or examination by the quality control unit before release for manufacturing or packaging;

(2) Holding rejected components, drug product containers, closures, and labeling before disposition;

(3) Storage of released components, drug product containers, closures, and labeling;

(4) Storage of in-process materials;

(5) Manufacturing and processing operations;

(6) Packaging and labeling operations;

(7) Quarantine storage before release of drug products;

(8) Storage of drug products after release;

(9) Control and laboratory operations;

(10) Aseptic processing, which includes as appropriate:

(i) Floors, walls, and ceilings of smooth, hard surfaces that are easily cleanable;

(ii) Temperature and humidity controls;

(iii) An air supply filtered through high-efficiency particulate air filters under positive pressure, regardless of whether flow is laminar or nonlaminar;

(iv) A system for monitoring environmental conditions;

(v) A system for cleaning and disinfecting the room and equipment to produce aseptic conditions;

(vi) A system for maintaining any equipment used to control the aseptic conditions.

(d) Operations relating to the manufacture, processing, and packing of penicillin shall be performed in facilities separate from those used for other drug products for human use.

[43 FR 45077, Sept. 29, 1978, as amended at 60 FR 4091, Jan. 20, 1995]

§211.44   Lighting.

Adequate lighting shall be provided in all areas.

§211.46   Ventilation, air filtration, air heating and cooling.

(a) Adequate ventilation shall be provided.

(b) Equipment for adequate control over air pressure, micro-organisms, dust, humidity, and temperature shall be provided when appropriate for the manufacture, processing, packing, or holding of a drug product.

(c) Air filtration systems, including prefilters and particulate matter air filters, shall be used when appropriate on air supplies to production areas. If air is recirculated to production areas, measures shall be taken to control recirculation of dust from production. In areas where air contamination occurs during production, there shall be adequate exhaust systems or other systems adequate to control contaminants.

(d) Air-handling systems for the manufacture, processing, and packing of penicillin shall be completely separate from those for other drug products for human use.

§211.48 Plumbing.

(a) Potable water shall be supplied under continuous positive pressure in a plumbing system free of defects that could contribute contamination to any drug product. Potable water shall meet the standards prescribed in the Environmental Protection Agency's Primary Drinking Water Regulations set forth in 40 CFR part 141. Water not meeting such standards shall not be permitted in the potable water system.

(b) Drains shall be of adequate size and, where connected directly to a sewer, shall be provided with an air break or other mechanical device to prevent back-siphonage.

[43 FR 45077, Sept. 29, 1978, as amended at 48 FR 11426, Mar. 18, 1983]

§211.50 Sewage and refuse.

Sewage, trash, and other refuse in and from the building and immediate premises shall be disposed of in a safe and sanitary manner.

§211.52 Washing and toilet facilities.

Adequate washing facilities shall be provided, including hot and cold water, soap or detergent, air driers or single-service towels, and clean toilet facilities easily accessible to working areas.

§211.56 Sanitation.

(a) Any building used in the manufacture, processing, packing, or holding of a drug product shall be maintained in a clean and sanitary condition, Any such building shall be free of infestation by rodents, birds, insects, and other vermin (other than laboratory animals). Trash and organic waste matter shall be held and disposed of in a timely and sanitary manner.

(b) There shall be written procedures assigning responsibility for sanitation and describing in sufficient detail the cleaning schedules, methods, equipment, and materials to be used in cleaning the buildings and facilities; such written procedures shall be followed.

(c) There shall be written procedures for use of suitable rodenticides, insecticides, fungicides, fumigating agents, and cleaning and sanitizing agents. Such written procedures shall be designed to prevent the contamination of equipment, components, drug product containers, closures, packaging, labeling materials, or drug products and shall be followed. Rodenticides, insecticides, and fungicides shall not be used unless registered and used in accordance with the Federal Insecticide, Fungicide, and Rodenticide Act (7 U.S.C. 135).

(d) Sanitation procedures shall apply to work performed by contractors or temporary employees as well as work performed by full-time employees during the ordinary course of operations.

§211.58   Maintenance.

Any building used in the manufacture, processing, packing, or holding of a drug product shall be maintained in a good state of repair.

Subpart D--Equipment

§211.63   Equipment design, size, and location.

Equipment used in the manufacture, processing, packing, or holding of a drug product shall be of appropriate design, adequate size, and suitably located to facilitate operations for its intended use and for its cleaning and maintenance.

§211.65   Equipment construction.

(a) Equipment shall be constructed so that surfaces that contact components, in-process materials, or drug products shall not be reactive, additive, or absorptive so as to alter the safety, identity, strength, quality, or purity of the drug product beyond the official or other established requirements.

(b) Any substances required for operation, such as lubricants or coolants, shall not come into contact with components, drug product containers, closures, in-process materials, or drug products so as to alter the safety, identity, strength, quality, or purity of the drug product beyond the official or other established requirements.

§211.67   Equipment cleaning and maintenance.

(a) Equipment and utensils shall be cleaned, maintained, and, as appropriate for the nature of the drug, sanitized and/or sterilized at appropriate intervals to prevent malfunctions or contamination that would alter the safety, identity, strength, quality, or purity of the drug product beyond the official or other established requirements.

(b) Written procedures shall be established and followed for cleaning and maintenance of equipment, including utensils, used in the manufacture, processing, packing, or holding of a drug product. These procedures shall include, but are not necessarily limited to, the following:

(1) Assignment of responsibility for cleaning and maintaining equipment;

(2) Maintenance and cleaning schedules, including, where appropriate, sanitizing schedules;

(3) A description in sufficient detail of the methods, equipment, and materials used in cleaning and maintenance operations, and the methods of disassembling and reassembling equipment as necessary to assure proper cleaning and maintenance;

(4) Removal or obliteration of previous batch identification;

(5) Protection of clean equipment from contamination prior to use;

(6) Inspection of equipment for cleanliness immediately before use.

(c) Records shall be kept of maintenance, cleaning, sanitizing, and inspection as specified in §§211.180 and 211.182.

[43 FR 45077, Sept. 29, 1978, as amended at 73 FR 51931, Sept. 8, 2008]

§211.68 Automatic, mechanical, and electronic equipment.

(a) Automatic, mechanical, or electronic equipment or other types of equipment, including computers, or related systems that will perform a function satisfactorily, may be used in the manufacture, processing, packing, and holding of a drug product. If such equipment is so used, it shall be routinely calibrated, inspected, or checked according to a written program designed to assure proper performance. Written records of those calibration checks and inspections shall be maintained.

(b) Appropriate controls shall be exercised over computer or related systems to assure that changes in master production and control records or other records are instituted only by authorized personnel. Input to and output from the computer or related system of formulas or other records or data shall be checked for accuracy. The degree and frequency of input/output verification shall be based on the complexity and reliability of the computer or related system. A backup file of data entered into the computer or related system shall be maintained except where certain data, such as calculations performed in connection with laboratory analysis, are eliminated by computerization or other automated processes. In such instances a written record of the program shall be maintained along with appropriate validation data. Hard copy or alternative systems, such as duplicates, tapes, or microfilm, designed to assure that backup data are exact and complete and that it is secure from alteration, inadvertent erasures, or loss shall be maintained.

(c) Such automated equipment used for performance of operations addressed by §§211.101(c) or (d), 211.103, 211.182, or 211.188(b)(11) can satisfy the requirements included in those sections relating to the performance of an operation by one person and checking by another person if such equipment is used in conformity with this section, and one person checks that the equipment properly performed the operation.

[43 FR 45077, Sept. 29, 1978, as amended at 60 FR 4091, Jan. 20, 1995; 73 FR 51932, Sept. 8, 2008]

§211.72   Filters.

Filters for liquid filtration used in the manufacture, processing, or packing of injectable drug products intended for human use shall not release fibers into such products. Fiber-releasing filters may be used when it is not possible to manufacture such products without the use of these filters. If use of a fiber-releasing filter is necessary, an additional nonfiber-releasing filter having a maximum nominal pore size rating of 0.2 micron (0.45 micron if the manufacturing conditions so dictate) shall subsequently be used to reduce the content of particles in the injectable drug product. The use of an asbestos-containing filter is prohibited.

[73 FR 51932, Sept. 8, 2008]

Subpart E--Control of Components and Drug Product Containers and Closures

§211.80   General requirements.

(a) There shall be written procedures describing in sufficient detail the receipt, identification, storage, handling, sampling, testing, and approval or rejection of components and drug product containers and closures; such written procedures shall be followed.

(b) Components and drug product containers and closures shall at all times be handled and stored in a manner to prevent contamination.

(c) Bagged or boxed components of drug product containers, or closures shall be stored off the floor and suitably spaced to permit cleaning and inspection.

(d) Each container or grouping of containers for components or drug product containers, or closures shall be identified with a distinctive code for each lot in each shipment received. This code shall be used in recording the disposition of each lot. Each lot shall be appropriately identified as to its status (i.e., quarantine, approved, or rejected).

§211.82 Receipt and storage of untested components, drug product containers, and closures.

(a) Upon receipt and before acceptance, each container or grouping of containers of components, drug product containers, and closures shall be examined visually for appropriate labeling as to contents, container damage or broken seals, and contamination.

(b) Components, drug product containers, and closures shall be stored under quarantine until they have been tested or examined, whichever is appropriate, and released. Storage within the area shall conform to the requirements of §211.80.

[43 FR 45077, Sept. 29, 1978, as amended at 73 FR 51932, Sept. 8, 2008]

§211.84 Testing and approval or rejection of components, drug product containers, and closures.

(a) Each lot of components, drug product containers, and closures shall be withheld from use until the lot has been sampled, tested, or examined, as appropriate, and released for use by the quality control unit.

(b) Representative samples of each shipment of each lot shall be collected for testing or examination. The number of containers to be sampled, and the amount of material to be taken from each container, shall be based upon appropriate criteria such as statistical criteria for component variability, confidence levels, and degree of precision desired, the past quality history of the supplier, and the quantity needed for analysis and reserve where required by §211.170.

(c) Samples shall be collected in accordance with the following procedures:

(1) The containers of components selected shall be cleaned when necessary in a manner to prevent introduction of contaminants into the component.

(2) The containers shall be opened, sampled, and resealed in a manner designed to prevent contamination of

their contents and contamination of other components, drug product containers, or closures.

(3) Sterile equipment and aseptic sampling techniques shall be used when necessary.

(4) If it is necessary to sample a component from the top, middle, and bottom of its container, such sample subdivisions shall not be composited for testing.

(5) Sample containers shall be identified so that the following information can be determined: name of the material sampled, the lot number, the container from which the sample was taken, the date on which the sample was taken, and the name of the person who collected the sample.

(6) Containers from which samples have been taken shall be marked to show that samples have been removed from them.

(d) Samples shall be examined and tested as follows:

(1) At least one test shall be conducted to verify the identity of each component of a drug product. Specific identity tests, if they exist, shall be used.

(2) Each component shall be tested for conformity with all appropriate written specifications for purity, strength, and quality. In lieu of such testing by the manufacturer, a report of analysis may be accepted from the supplier of a component, provided that at least one specific identity test is conducted on such component by the manufacturer, and provided that the manufacturer establishes the reliability of the supplier's analyses through appropriate validation of the supplier's test results at appropriate intervals.

(3) Containers and closures shall be tested for conformity with all appropriate written specifications. In lieu of such testing by the manufacturer, a certificate of testing may be accepted from the supplier, provided that at least a visual identification is conducted on such containers/closures by the manufacturer and provided that the manufacturer establishes the reliability of the supplier's test results through appropriate validation of the supplier's test results at appropriate intervals.

(4) When appropriate, components shall be microscopically examined.

(5) Each lot of a component, drug product container, or closure that is liable to contamination with filth, insect infestation, or other extraneous adulterant shall be examined against established specifications for such contamination.

(6) Each lot of a component, drug product container, or closure with potential for microbiological contamination that is objectionable in view of its intended use shall be subjected to microbiological tests before use.

(e) Any lot of components, drug product containers, or closures that meets the appropriate written specifications of identity, strength, quality, and purity and related tests under paragraph (d) of this section may be approved and released for use. Any lot of such material that does not meet such specifications shall be rejected.

[43 FR 45077, Sept. 29, 1978, as amended at 63 FR 14356, Mar. 25, 1998; 73 FR 51932, Sept. 8, 2008]

§211.86   Use of approved components, drug product containers, and closures.

Components, drug product containers, and closures approved for use shall be rotated so that the oldest approved stock is used first. Deviation from this requirement is permitted if such deviation is temporary and appropriate.

§211.87   Retesting of approved components, drug product containers, and closures.

Components, drug product containers, and closures shall be retested or reexamined, as appropriate, for identity, strength, quality, and purity and approved or rejected by the quality control unit in accordance with §211.84 as necessary, e.g., after storage for long periods or after exposure to air, heat or other conditions that might adversely affect the component, drug product container, or closure.

§211.89   Rejected components, drug product containers, and closures.

Rejected components, drug product containers, and closures shall be identified and controlled under a quarantine system designed to prevent their use in manufacturing or processing operations for which they are unsuitable.

§211.94   Drug product containers and closures.

(a) Drug product containers and closures shall not be reactive, additive, or absorptive so as to alter the safety, identity, strength, quality, or purity of the drug beyond the official or established requirements.

(b) Container closure systems shall provide adequate protection against foreseeable external factors in storage and use that can cause deterioration or contamination of the drug product.

(c) Drug product containers and closures shall be clean and, where indicated by the nature of the drug, sterilized and processed to remove pyrogenic properties to assure that they are suitable for their intended use. Such depyrogenation processes shall be validated.

(d) Standards or specifications, methods of testing, and, where indicated, methods of cleaning, sterilizing, and processing to remove pyrogenic properties shall be written and followed for drug product containers and closures.

(e) *Medical gas containers and closures must meet the following requirements*--(1) Gas-specific use outlet connections. Portable cryogenic medical gas containers that are not manufactured with permanent gas use outlet connections (*e.g.*, those that have been silver-brazed) must have gas-specific use outlet connections that are attached to the valve body so that they cannot be readily removed or replaced (without making the valve inoperable and preventing the containers' use) except by the manufacturer. For the purposes of this paragraph, the term "manufacturer" includes any individual or firm that fills high-pressure medical gas cylinders or cryogenic medical gas containers. For the purposes of this section, a "portable cryogenic medical gas container" is one that is capable of being transported and is intended to be attached to a medical gas supply system within a hospital, health care entity, nursing home, other facility, or home health care setting, or is a base unit used to fill small cryogenic gas containers for use by individual patients. The term does not include cryogenic containers that are not designed to be connected to a medical gas supply system, *e.g.*, tank trucks, trailers, rail cars, or small cryogenic gas containers for use by individual patients (including portable liquid oxygen units as defined at §868.5655 of this chapter).

(2) *Label and coloring requirements.* The labeling specified at §201.328(a) of this chapter must be affixed to the container in a manner that does not interfere with other labeling and such that it is not susceptible to becoming worn or inadvertently detached during normal use. Each such label as well as materials used for coloring medical gas containers must be reasonably resistant to fading, durable when exposed to atmospheric conditions, and not readily soluble in water.

[43 FR 45077, Sept. 29, 1978, as amended at 73 FR 51932, Sept. 8, 2008; 81 FR 81697, January 17, 2017]

Subpart F--Production and Process Controls
§211.100 Written procedures; deviations.

(a) There shall be written procedures for production and process control designed to assure that the drug products have the identity, strength, quality, and purity they purport or are represented to possess. Such procedures shall include all requirements in this subpart. These written procedures, including any changes, shall be drafted, reviewed, and approved by the appropriate organizational units and reviewed and approved by the quality control unit.

(b) Written production and process control procedures shall be followed in the execution of the various production and process control functions and shall be documented at the time of performance. Any deviation from the written procedures shall be recorded and justified.

§211.101 Charge-in of components.

Written production and control procedures shall include the following, which are designed to assure that the drug products produced have the identity, strength, quality, and purity they purport or are represented to possess:

(a) The batch shall be formulated with the intent to provide not less than 100 percent of the labeled or established amount of active ingredient.

(b) Components for drug product manufacturing shall be weighed, measured, or subdivided as appropriate. If a component is removed from the original container to another, the new container shall be identified with the following information:

(1) Component name or item code;

(2) Receiving or control number;

(3) Weight or measure in new container;

(4) Batch for which component was dispensed, including its product name, strength, and lot number.

(c) Weighing, measuring, or subdividing operations for components shall be adequately supervised. Each container of component dispensed to manufacturing shall be examined by a second person to assure that:

(1) The component was released by the quality control unit;

(2) The weight or measure is correct as stated in the batch production records;

(3) The containers are properly identified. If the weighing, measuring, or subdividing operations are performed by automated equipment under §211.68, only one person is needed to assure paragraphs (c)(1), (c)(2), and (c)(3) of this section.

(d) Each component shall either be added to the batch by one person and verified by a second person or, if the components are added by automated equipment under §211.68, only verified by one person.

[43 FR 45077, Sept. 29, 1978, as amended at 73 FR 51932, Sept. 8, 2008]

§211.103   Calculation of yield.

Actual yields and percentages of theoretical yield shall be determined at the conclusion of each appropriate phase of manufacturing, processing, packaging, or holding of the drug product. Such calculations shall either be performed by one person and independently verified by a second person, or, if the yield is calculated by automated equipment under § 211.68, be independently verified by one person.

[73 FR 51932, Sept. 8, 2008]

§211.105   Equipment identification.

(a) All compounding and storage containers, processing lines, and major equipment used during the production of a batch of a drug product shall be properly identified at all times to indicate their contents and, when necessary, the phase of processing of the batch.

(b) Major equipment shall be identified by a distinctive identification number or code that shall be recorded in the batch production record to show the specific equipment used in the manufacture of each batch of a drug product. In cases where only one of a particular type of equipment exists in a manufacturing facility, the name of the equipment may be used in lieu of a distinctive identification number or code.

§211.110   Sampling and testing of in-process materials and drug products.

(a) To assure batch uniformity and integrity of drug products, written procedures shall be established and followed that describe the in-process controls, and tests, or examinations to be conducted on appropriate samples of in-process materials of each batch. Such control procedures shall be established to monitor the output and to validate the performance of those manufacturing processes that may be responsible for causing variability in the characteristics of in-process material and the drug product. Such control procedures shall include, but are not limited to, the following, where appropriate:

(1) Tablet or capsule weight variation;
(2) Disintegration time;
(3) Adequacy of mixing to assure uniformity and homogeneity;
(4) Dissolution time and rate;
(5) Clarity, completeness, or pH of solutions.
(6) Bioburden testing.

(b) Valid in-process specifications for such characteristics shall be consistent with drug product final specifications and shall be derived from previous acceptable process average and process variability estimates where possible and determined by the application of suitable statistical procedures where appropriate. Examination and testing of samples shall assure that the drug product and in-process material conform to specifications.

(c) In-process materials shall be tested for identity, strength, quality, and purity as appropriate, and approved or rejected by the quality control unit, during the production process, e.g., at commencement or completion of significant phases or after storage for long periods.

(d) Rejected in-process materials shall be identified and controlled under a quarantine system designed to prevent their use in manufacturing or processing operations for which thoy aro unsuitable.

[43 FR 45077, Sept. 29, 1978, as amended at 73 FR 51932, Sept. 8, 2008]

§211.111   Time limitations on production.

When appropriate, time limits for the completion of each phase of production shall be established to assure the quality of the drug product. Deviation from established time limits may be acceptable if such deviation does not compromise the quality of the drug product. Such deviation shall be justified and documented.

§211.113   Control of microbiological contamination.

(a) Appropriate written procedures, designed to prevent objectionable microorganisms in drug products not required to be sterile, shall be established and followed.

(b) Appropriate written procedures, designed to prevent microbiological contamination of drug products purporting to be sterile, shall be established and followed. Such procedures shall include validation of all aseptic and sterilization processes.

[43 FR 45077, Sept. 29, 1978, as amended at 73 FR 51932, Sept. 8, 2008]

§211.115   Reprocessing.

(a) Written procedures shall be established and followed prescribing a system for reprocessing batches that do not conform to standards or specifications and the steps to be taken to insure that the reprocessed batches will conform with all established standards, specifications, and characteristics.

(b) Reprocessing shall not be performed without the review and approval of the quality control unit.

Subpart G--Packaging and Labeling Control

§211.122   Materials examination and usage criteria.

(a) There shall be written procedures describing in sufficient detail the receipt, identification, storage, handling, sampling, examination, and/or testing of labeling and packaging materials; such written procedures shall be followed. Labeling and packaging materials shall be representatively sampled, and examined or tested upon receipt and before use in packaging or labeling of a drug product.

(b) Any labeling or packaging materials meeting appropriate written specifications may be approved and released for use. Any labeling or packaging materials that do not meet such specifications shall be rejected to prevent their use in operations for which they are unsuitable.

(c) Records shall be maintained for each shipment received of each different labeling and packaging material indicating receipt, examination or testing, and whether accepted or rejected.

(d) Labels and other labeling materials for each different drug product, strength, dosage form, or quantity of contents shall be stored separately with suitable identification. Access to the storage area shall be limited to authorized personnel.

(e) Obsolete and outdated labels, labeling, and other packaging materials shall be destroyed.

(f) Use of gang-printed labeling for different drug products, or different strengths or net contents of the same drug product, is prohibited unless the labeling from gang-printed sheets is adequately differentiated by size, shape, or color.

(g) If cut labeling is used for immediate container labels, individual unit cartons, or multiunit cartons containing immediate containers that are not packaged in individual unit cartons, packaging and labeling operations shall include one of the following special control procedures:

(1) Dedication of labeling and packaging lines to each different strength of each different drug product;

(2) Use of appropriate electronic or electromechanical equipment to conduct a 100-percent examination for correct labeling during or after completion of finishing operations; or

(3) Use of visual inspection to conduct a 100-percent examination for correct labeling during or after completion of finishing operations for hand-applied labeling. Such examination shall be performed by one person and independently verified by a second person.

(4) Use of any automated technique, including differentiation by labeling size and shape, that physically prevents incorrect labeling from being processed by labeling and packaging equipment.

(h) Printing devices on, or associated with, manufacturing lines used to imprint labeling upon the drug product unit label or case shall be monitored to assure that all imprinting conforms to the print specified in the batch production record.

[43 FR 45077, Sept. 29, 1978, as amended at 58 FR 41353, Aug. 3, 1993; 77 FR 16163, Mar. 20, 2012]

§211.125 Labeling issuance.

(a) Strict control shall be exercised over labeling issued for use in drug product labeling operations.

(b) Labeling materials issued for a batch shall be carefully examined for identity and conformity to the labeling specified in the master or batch production records.

(c) Procedures shall be used to reconcile the quantities of labeling issued, used, and returned, and shall require evaluation of discrepancies found between the quantity of drug product finished and the quantity of labeling issued when such discrepancies are outside narrow preset limits based on historical operating data. Such discrepancies shall be investigated in accordance with §211.192. Labeling reconciliation is waived for cut or roll labeling if a 100-percent examination for correct labeling is performed in accordance with §211.122(g)(2). Labeling reconciliation is also waived for 360° wraparound labels on portable cryogenic medical gas containers.

(d) All excess labeling bearing lot or control numbers shall be destroyed.

(e) Returned labeling shall be maintained and stored in a manner to prevent mixups and provide proper identification.

(f) Procedures shall be written describing in sufficient detail the control procedures employed for the issuance of labeling; such written procedures shall be followed.

[43 FR 45077, Sept. 29, 1978, as amended at 58 FR 41354, Aug. 3, 1993; 81 FR 81697, January 17, 2017]

§211.130 Packaging and labeling operations.

There shall be written procedures designed to assure that correct labels, labeling, and packaging materials are used for drug products; such written procedures shall be followed. These procedures shall incorporate the following features:

(a) Prevention of mixups and cross-contamination by physical or spatial separation from operations on other drug products.

(b) Identification and handling of filled drug product containers that are set aside and held in unlabeled condition for future labeling operations to preclude mislabeling of individual containers, lots, or portions of lots.

Identification need not be applied to each individual container but shall be sufficient to determine name, strength, quantity of contents, and lot or control number of each container.

(c) Identification of the drug product with a lot or control number that permits determination of the history of the manufacture and control of the batch.

(d) Examination of packaging and labeling materials for suitability and correctness before packaging operations, and documentation of such examination in the batch production record.

(e) Inspection of the packaging and labeling facilities immediately before use to assure that all drug products have been removed from previous operations. Inspection shall also be made to assure that packaging and labeling materials not suitable for subsequent operations have been removed. Results of inspection shall be documented in the batch production records.

[43 FR 45077, Sept. 29, 197? amended at 58 FR 41354, Aug. 3, 1993]

§211.132 Tamper-evident packaging requirements for over-the-counter (OTC) human drug products.

(a) *General.* The Food and Drug Administration has the authority under the Federal Food, Drug, and Cosmetic Act (the act) to establish a uniform national requirement for tamper-evident packaging of OTC drug products that will improve the security of OTC drug packaging and help assure the safety and effectiveness of OTC drug products. An OTC drug product (except a dermatological, dentifrice, insulin, or lozenge product) for retail sale that is not packaged in a tamper-resistant package or that is not properly labeled under this section is adulterated under section 501 of the act or misbranded under section 502 of the act, or both.

(b) *Requirements for tamper-evident package.* (1) Each manufacturer and packer who packages an OTC drug product (except a dermatological, dentifrice, insulin, or lozenge product) for retail sale shall package the product in a tamper-evident package, if this product is accessible to the public while held for sale. A tamper-evident package is one having one or more indicators or barriers to entry which, if breached or missing, can reasonably be expected to provide visible evidence to consumers that tampering has occurred. To reduce the likelihood of successful tampering and to increase the likelihood that consumers will discover if a product has been tampered with, the package is required to be distinctive by design or by the use of one or more indicators or barriers to entry that employ an identifying characteristic (e.g., a pattern, name, registered trademark, logo, or picture). For purposes of this section, the term "distinctive by design" means the packaging cannot be duplicated with commonly available materials or through commonly available processes. A tamper-evident package may involve an immediate-container and closure system or secondary-container or carton system or any combination of systems intended to provide a visual indication of package integrity. The tamper-evident feature shall be designed to and shall remain intact when handled in a reasonable manner during manufacture, distribution, and retail display.

(2) In addition to the tamper-evident packaging feature described in paragraph (b)(1) of this section, any two-piece, hard gelatin capsule covered by this section must be sealed using an acceptable tamper-evident technology.

(c) *Labeling.* (1) In order to alert consumers to the specific tamper-evident feature(s) used, each retail package of an OTC drug product covered by this section (except ammonia inhalant in crushable glass ampules, containers ofcompressed medical oxygen, or aerosol products that depend upon the power of a liquefied or compressed gas to expel the contents from the container) is required to bear a statement that:

(i) Identifies all tamper-evident feature(s) and any capsule sealing technologies used to comply with paragraph (b) of this section;

(ii) Is prominently placed on the package; and

(iii) Is so placed that it will be unaffected if the tamper-evident feature of the package is breached or missing.

(2) If the tamper-evident feature chosen to meet the requirements in paragraph (b) of this section uses an identifying characteristic, that characteristic is required to

be referred to in the labeling statement. For example, the labeling statement on a bottle with a shrink band could say "For your protection, this bottle has an imprinted seal around the neck."

(d) *Request for exemptions from packaging and labeling requirements.* A manufacturer or packer may request an exemption from the packaging and labeling requirements of this section. A request for an exemption is required to be submitted in the form of a citizen petition under §10.30 of this chapter and should be clearly identified on the envelope as a "Request for Exemption from the Tamper-Evident Packaging Rule." The petition is required to contain the following:

(1) The name of the drug product or, if the petition seeks an exemption for a drug class, the name of the drug class, and a list of products within that class.

(2) The reasons that the drug product's compliance with the tamper-evident packaging or labeling requirements of this section is unnecessary or cannot be achieved.

(3) A description of alternative steps that are available, or that the petitioner has already taken, to reduce the likelihood that the product or drug class will be the subject of malicious adulteration.

(4) Other information justifying an exemption.

(e) *OTC drug products subject to approved new drug applications.* Holders of approved new drug applications for OTC drug products are required under §314.70 of this chapter to provide the agency with notification of changes in packaging and labeling to comply with the requirements of this section. Changes in packaging and labeling required by this regulation may be made before FDA approval, as provided under §314.70(c) of this chapter. Manufacturing changes by which capsules are to be sealed require prior FDA approval under §314.70(b) of this chapter.

(f) *Poison Prevention Packaging Act of 1970.* This section does not affect any requirements for "special packaging" as defined under §310.3(l) of this chapter and required under the Poison Prevention Packaging Act of 1970. (Approved by the Office of Management and Budget under OMB control number 0910-0149)

[54 FR 5228, Feb. 2, 1989, as amended at 63 FR 59470, Nov. 4, 1998]

§211.134   Drug product inspection.

(a) Packaged and labeled products shall be examined during finishing operations to provide assurance that containers and packages in the lot have the correct label.

(b) A representative sample of units shall be collected at the completion of finishing operations and shall be visually examined for correct labeling.

(c) Results of these examinations shall be recorded in the batch production or control records.

§211.137   Expiration dating.

(a) To assure that a drug product meets applicable standards of identity, strength, quality, and purity at the time of use, it shall bear an expiration date determined by appropriate stability testing described in §211.166.

(b) Expiration dates shall be related to any storage conditions stated on the labeling, as determined by stability studies described in §211.166.

(c) If the drug product is to be reconstituted at the time of dispensing, its labeling shall bear expiration information for both the reconstituted and unreconstituted drug products.

(d) Expiration dates shall appear on labeling in accordance with the requirements of §201.17 of this chapter.

(e) Homeopathic drug products shall be exempt from the requirements of this section.

(f) Allergenic extracts that are labeled "No U.S. Standard of Potency" are exempt from the requirements of this section.

(g) New drug products for investigational use are exempt from the requirements of this section, provided that they meet appropriate standards or specifications as demonstrated by stability studies during their use in clinical investigations. Where new drug products for investigational use are to be reconstituted at the time of dispensing, their labeling shall bear expiration information for the reconstituted drug product.

(h) Pending consideration of a proposed exemption, published in the FEDERAL REGISTER of September 29,

1978, the requirements in this section shall not be enforced for human OTC drug products if their labeling does not bear dosage limitations and they are stable for at least 3 years as supported by appropriate stability data.

[43 FR 45077, Sept. 29, 1978, as amended at 46 FR 56412, Nov. 17, 1981; 60 FR 4091, Jan. 20, 1995]

Subpart H--Holding and Distribution

§211.142   Warehousing procedures.

Written procedures describing the warehousing of drug products shall be established and followed. They shall include:

(a) Quarantine of drug products before release by the quality control unit.

(b) Storage of drug products under appropriate conditions of temperature, humidity, and light so that the identity, strength, quality, and purity of the drug products are not affected.

§211.150   Distribution procedures.

Written procedures shall be established, and followed, describing the distribution of drug products. They shall include:

(a) A procedure whereby the oldest approved stock of a drug product is distributed first. Deviation from this requirement is permitted if such deviation is temporary and appropriate.

(b) A system by which the distribution of each lot of drug product can be readily determined to facilitate its recall if necessary.

Subpart I--Laboratory Controls

§211.160   General requirements.

(a) The establishment of any specifications, standards, sampling plans, test procedures, or other laboratory control mechanisms required by this subpart, including any change in such specifications, standards, sampling plans, test procedures, or other laboratory control mechanisms, shall be drafted by the appropriate organizational unit and reviewed and approved by the quality control unit. The requirements in this subpart shall be followed and shall be documented at the time of performance. Any deviation from the written specifications, standards, sampling plans, test procedures, or other laboratory control mechanisms shall be recorded and justified.

(b) Laboratory controls shall include the establishment of scientifically sound and appropriate specifications, standards, sampling plans, and test procedures designed to assure that components, drug product containers, closures, in-process materials, labeling, and drug products conform to appropriate standards of identity, strength, quality, and purity. Laboratory controls shall include:

(1) Determination of conformity to applicable written specifications for the acceptance of each lot within each shipment of components, drug product containers, closures, and labeling used in the manufacture, processing, packing, or holding of drug products. The specifications shall include a description of the sampling and testing procedures used. Samples shall be representative and adequately identified. Such procedures shall also require appropriate retesting of any component, drug product container, or closure that is subject to deterioration.

(2) Determination of conformance to written specifications and a description of sampling and testing procedures for in-process materials. Such samples shall be representative and properly identified.

(3) Determination of conformance to written descriptions of sampling procedures and appropriate specifications for drug products. Such samples shall be representative and properly identified.

(4) The calibration of instruments, apparatus, gauges, and recording devices at suitable intervals in accordance with an established written program containing specific directions, schedules, limits for accuracy and precision, and provisions for remedial action in the event accuracy and/or precision limits are not met. Instruments, apparatus, gauges, and recording devices not meeting established specifications shall not be used.

[43 FR 45077, Sept. 29, 1978, as amended at 73 FR 51932, Sept. 8, 2008]

§211.165 Testing and release for distribution.

(a) For each batch of drug product, there shall be appropriate laboratory determination of satisfactory conformance to final specifications for the drug product, including the identity and strength of each active ingredient, prior to release. Where sterility and/or pyrogen testing are conducted on specific batches of shortlived radiopharmaceuticals, such batches may be released prior to completion of sterility and/or pyrogen testing, provided such testing is completed as soon as possible.

(b) There shall be appropriate laboratory testing, as necessary, of each batch of drug product required to be free of objectionable microorganisms.

(c) Any sampling and testing plans shall be described in written procedures that shall include the method of sampling and the number of units per batch to be tested; such written procedure shall be followed.

(d) Acceptance criteria for the sampling and testing conducted by the quality control unit shall be adequate to assure that batches of drug products meet each appropriate specification and appropriate statistical quality control criteria as a condition for their approval and release. The statistical quality control criteria shall include appropriate acceptance levels and/or appropriate rejection levels.

(e) The accuracy, sensitivity, specificity, and reproducibility of test methods employed by the firm shall be established and documented. Such validation and documentation may be accomplished in accordance with §211.194(a)(2).

(f) Drug products failing to meet established standards or specifications and any other relevant quality control criteria shall be rejected. Reprocessing may be performed. Prior to acceptance and use, reprocessed material must meet appropriate standards, specifications, and any other relevant criteria.

§211.166   Stability testing.

(a) There shall be a written testing program designed to assess the stability characteristics of drug products. The results of such stability testing shall be used in determining appropriate storage conditions and expiration dates. The written program shall be followed and shall include:

(1) Sample size and test intervals based on statistical criteria for each attribute examined to assure valid estimates of stability;

(2) Storage conditions for samples retained for testing;

(3) Reliable, meaningful, and specific test methods;

(4) Testing of the drug product in the same container-closure system as that in which the drug product is marketed;

(5) Testing of drug products for reconstitution at the time of dispensing (as directed in the labeling) as well as after they are reconstituted.

(b) An adequate number of batches of each drug product shall be tested to determine an appropriate expiration date and a record of such data shall be maintained. Accelerated studies, combined with basic stability information on the components, drug products, and container-closure system, may be used to support tentative expiration dates provided full shelf life studies are not available and are being conducted. Where data from accelerated studies are used to project a tentative expiration date that is beyond a date supported by actual shelf life studies, there must be stability studies conducted, including drug product testing at appropriate intervals, until the tentative expiration date is verified or the appropriate expiration date determined.

(c) For homeopathic drug products, the requirements of this section are as follows:

(1) There shall be a written assessment of stability based at least on testing or examination of the drug product for compatibility of the ingredients, and based on marketing experience with the drug product to indicate that there is no degradation of the product for the normal or expected period of use.

(2) Evaluation of stability shall be based on the same container-closure system in which the drug product is being marketed.

(d) Allergenic extracts that are labeled "No U.S. Standard of Potency" are exempt from the requirements of this section.

[43 FR 45077, Sept. 29, 1978, as amended at 46 FR 56412, Nov. 17, 1981]

§211.167   Special testing requirements.

(a) For each batch of drug product purporting to be sterile and/or pyrogen-free, there shall be appropriate laboratory testing to determine conformance to such requirements. The test procedures shall be in writing and shall be followed.

(b) For each batch of ophthalmic ointment, there shall be appropriate testing to determine conformance to specifications regarding the presence of foreign particles and harsh or abrasive substances. The test procedures shall be in writing and shall be followed.

(c) For each batch of controlled-release dosage form, there shall be appropriate laboratory testing to determine conformance to the specifications for the rate of release of each active ingredient. The test procedures shall be in writing and shall be followed.

§211.170   Reserve samples.

(a) An appropriately identified reserve sample that is representative of each lot in each shipment of each active ingredient shall be retained. The reserve sample consists of at least twice the quantity necessary for all tests required to determine whether the active ingredient meets its established specifications, except for sterility and pyrogen testing. The retention time is as follows:

(1) For an active ingredient in a drug product other than those described in paragraphs (a) (2) and (3) of this section, the reserve sample shall be retained for 1 year after the expiration date of the last lot of the drug product containing the active ingredient.

(2) For an active ingredient in a radioactive drug product, except for nonradioactive reagent kits, the reserve sample shall be retained for:

(i) Three months after the expiration date of the last lot of the drug product containing the active ingredient if the expiration dating period of the drug product is 30 days or less; or

(ii) Six months after the expiration date of the last lot of the drug product containing the active ingredient if the expiration dating period of the drug product is more than 30 days.

(3) For an active ingredient in an OTC drug product that is exempt from bearing an expiration date under §211.137, the reserve sample shall be retained for 3 years after distribution of the last lot of the drug product containing the active ingredient.

(b) An appropriately identified reserve sample that is representative of each lot or batch of drug product shall be retained and stored under conditions consistent with product labeling. The reserve sample shall be stored in the same immediate container-closure system in which the drug product is marketed or in one that has essentially the same characteristics. The reserve sample consists of at least twice the quantity necessary to perform all the required tests, except those for sterility and pyrogens. Except for those for drug products described in paragraph (b)(2) of this section, reserve samples from representative sample lots or batches selected by acceptable statistical procedures shall be examined visually at least once a year for evidence of deterioration unless visual examination would affect the integrity of the reserve sample. Any evidence of reserve sample deterioration shall be investigated in accordance with §211.192. The results of the examination shall be recorded and maintained with other stability data on the drug product. Reserve samples of compressed medical gases need not be retained. The retention time is as follows:

(1) For a drug product other than those described in paragraphs (b) (2) and (3) of this section, the reserve sample shall be retained for 1 year after the expiration date of the drug product.

(2) For a radioactive drug product, except for nonradioactive reagent kits, the reserve sample shall be retained for:

(i) Three months after the expiration date of the drug product if the expiration dating period of the drug product is 30 days or less; or

(ii) Six months after the expiration date of the drug product if the expiration dating period of the drug product is more than 30 days.

(3) For an OTC drug product that is exempt for bearing an expiration date under §211.137, the reserve sample must be retained for 3 years after the lot or batch of drug product is distributed.

[48 FR 13025, Mar. 29, 1983, as amended at 60 FR 4091, Jan. 20, 1995]

§211.173   Laboratory animals.

Animals used in testing components, in-process materials, or drug products for compliance with established specifications shall be maintained and controlled in a manner that assures their suitability for their intended use. They shall be identified, and adequate records shall be maintained showing the history of their use.

§211.176   Penicillin contamination.

If a reasonable possibility exists that a non-penicillin drug product has been exposed to cross-contamination with penicillin, the non-penicillin drug product shall be tested for the presence of penicillin. Such drug product shall not be marketed if detectable levels are found when tested according to procedures specified in 'Procedures for Detecting and Measuring Penicillin Contamination in Drugs,' which is incorporated by reference. Copies are available from the Division of Research and Testing (HFD-470), Center for Drug Evaluation and Research, Food and Drug Administration, 5001 Campus Dr.., College Park, MD 20740, or available for inspection at the National Archives and Records Administration (NARA). For information on the availability of this material at NARA, call 202-741-6030, or go to:
http://www.archives.gov/federal_register/code_of_feder al_regulations/ibr_locations.html.

[43 FR 45077, Sept. 29, 1978, as amended at 47 FR 9396, Mar. 5, 1982; 50 FR 8996, Mar. 6, 1985; 55 FR 11577, Mar. 29, 1990; 66 FR 56035, Nov. 6, 2001; 69 FR 18803, Apr. 9, 2004; 81 FR 49897, July 29, 2016]

Subpart J--Records and Reports

§211.180   General requirements.

(a) Any production, control, or distribution record that is required to be maintained in compliance with this part and is specifically associated with a batch of a drug product shall be retained for at least 1 year after the expiration date of the batch or, in the case of certain OTC drug products lacking expiration dating because they meet the criteria for exemption under §211.137, 3 years after distribution of the batch.

(b) Records shall be maintained for all components, drug product containers, closures, and labeling for at least 1 year after the expiration date or, in the case of certain OTC drug products lacking expiration dating because they meet the criteria for exemption under §211.137, 3 years after distribution of the last lot of drug product incorporating the component or using the container, closure, or labeling.

(c) All records required under this part, or copies of such records, shall be readily available for authorized inspection during the retention period at the establishment where the activities described in such records occurred. These records or copies thereof shall be subject to photocopying or other means of reproduction as part of such inspection. Records that can be immediately retrieved from another location by computer or other electronic means shall be considered as meeting the requirements of this paragraph.

(d) Records required under this part may be retained either as original records or as true copies such as photocopies, microfilm, microfiche, or other accurate reproductions of the original records. Where reduction techniques, such as microfilming, are used, suitable reader and photocopying equipment shall be readily available.

(e) Written records required by this part shall be maintained so that data therein can be used for evaluating, at least annually, the quality standards of each drug product to determine the need for changes in drug product specifications or manufacturing or control procedures. Written procedures shall be established and followed for such evaluations and shall include provisions for:

(1) A review of a representative number of batches, whether approved or rejected, and, where applicable, records associated with the batch.

(2) A review of complaints, recalls, returned or salvaged drug products, and investigations conducted under §211.192 for each drug product.

(f) Procedures shall be established to assure that the responsible officials of the firm, if they are not personally involved in or immediately aware of such actions, are notified in writing of any investigations conducted under §§211.198, 211.204, or 211.208 of these regulations, any recalls, reports of inspectional observations issued by the Food and Drug Administration, or any regulatory actions relating to good manufacturing practices brought by the Food and Drug Administration.

[43 FR 45077, Sept. 29, 1978, as amended at 60 FR 4091, Jan. 20, 1995]

§211.182   Equipment cleaning and use log.

A written record of major equipment cleaning, maintenance (except routine maintenance such as lubrication and adjustments), and use shall be included in individual equipment logs that show the date, time, product, and lot number of each batch processed. If equipment is dedicated to manufacture of one product, then individual equipment logs are not required, provided that lots or batches of such product follow in numerical order and are manufactured in numerical sequence. In cases where dedicated equipment is employed, the records of cleaning, maintenance, and use shall be part of the batch record. The persons performing and double-checking the cleaning and maintenance (or, if the cleaning and maintenance is performed using automated equipment under §211.68, just the person verifying the cleaning and maintenance done by the automated equipment) shall date and sign or initial the log indicating that the work was performed. Entries in the log shall be in chronological order.

§211.184 Component, drug product container, closure, and labeling records.

These records shall include the following:

(a) The identity and quantity of each shipment of each lot of components, drug product containers, closures, and labeling; the name of the supplier; the supplier's lot number(s) if known; the receiving code as specified in §211.80; and the date of receipt. The name and location of the prime manufacturer, if different from the supplier, shall be listed if known.

(b) The results of any test or examination performed (including those performed as required by §211.82(a), §211.84(d), or §211.122(a)) and the conclusions derived therefrom.

(c) An individual inventory record of each component, drug product container, and closure and, for each component, a reconciliation of the use of each lot of such component. The inventory record shall contain sufficient information to allow determination of any batch or lot of drug product associated with the use of each component, drug product container, and closure.

(d) Documentation of the examination and review of labels and labeling for conformity with established specifications in accord with §§211.122(c) and 211.130(c).

(e) The disposition of rejected components, drug product containers, closure, and labeling.

§211.186 Master production and control records.

(a) To assure uniformity from batch to batch, master production and control records for each drug product, including each batch size thereof, shall be prepared, dated, and signed (full signature, handwritten) by one person and independently checked, dated, and signed by a second person. The preparation of master production and control records shall be described in a written procedure and such written procedure shall be followed.

(b) Master production and control records shall include:

(1) The name and strength of the product and a description of the dosage form;

(2) The name and weight or measure of each active ingredient per dosage unit or per unit of weight or measure of the drug product, and a statement of the total weight or measure of any dosage unit;

(3) A complete list of components designated by names or codes sufficiently specific to indicate any special quality characteristic;

(4) An accurate statement of the weight or measure of each component, using the same weight system (metric, avoirdupois, or apothecary) for each component. Reasonable variations may be permitted, however, in the amount of components necessary for the preparation in the dosage form, provided they are justified in the master production and control records;

(5) A statement concerning any calculated excess of component;

(6) A statement of theoretical weight or measure at appropriate phases of processing;

(7) A statement of theoretical yield, including the maximum and minimum percentages of theoretical yield beyond which investigation according to §211.192 is required;

(8) A description of the drug product containers, closures, and packaging materials, including a specimen or copy of each label and all other labeling signed and dated by the person or persons responsible for approval of such labeling;

(9) Complete manufacturing and control instructions, sampling and testing procedures, specifications, special notations, and precautions to be followed.

§211.188   Batch production and control records.

Batch production and control records shall be prepared for each batch of drug product produced and shall include complete information relating to the production and control of each batch. These records shall include:

(a) An accurate reproduction of the appropriate master production or control record, checked for accuracy, dated, and signed;

(b) Documentation that each significant step in the manufacture, processing, packing, or holding of the batch was accomplished, including:

(1) Dates;

(2) Identity of individual major equipment and lines used;

(3) Specific identification of each batch of component or in-process material used;

(4) Weights and measures of components used in the course of processing;

(5) In-process and laboratory control results;

(6) Inspection of the packaging and labeling area before and after use;

(7) A statement of the actual yield and a statement of the percentage of theoretical yield at appropriate phases of processing;

(8) Complete labeling control records, including specimens or copies of all labeling used;

(9) Description of drug product containers and closures;

(10) Any sampling performed;

(11) Identification of the persons performing and directly supervising or checking each significant step in the operation, or if a significant step in the operation is performed by automated equipment under §211.68, the identification of the person checking the significant step performed by the automated equipment.

(12) Any investigation made according to §211.192.

(13) Results of examinations made in accordance with §211.134.

[43 FR 45077, Sept. 29, 1978, as amended at 73 FR 51933, Sept. 8, 2008]

§211.192   Production record review.

All drug product production and control records, including those for packaging and labeling, shall be reviewed and approved by the quality control unit to determine compliance with all established, approved written procedures before a batch is released or distributed. Any unexplained discrepancy (including a percentage of theoretical yield exceeding the maximum or minimum percentages established in master production and control records) or the failure of a batch or any of its components to meet any of its specifications shall be thoroughly investigated, whether or not the batch has already been distributed. The investigation shall extend to other batches of the same drug product and other drug products that may have been associated with the specific failure or discrepancy. A written record of the investigation shall be made and shall include the conclusions and follow up.

§211.194   Laboratory records.

(a) Laboratory records shall include complete data derived from all tests necessary to assure compliance with established specifications and standards, including examinations and assays, as follows:

(1) A description of the sample received for testing with identification of source (that is, location from where sample was obtained), quantity, lot number or other distinctive code, date sample was taken, and date sample was received for testing.

(2) A statement of each method used in the testing of the sample. The statement shall indicate the location of data that establish that the methods used in the testing of the sample meet proper standards of accuracy and reliability as applied to the product tested. (If the method employed is in the current revision of the United States Pharmacopeia, National Formulary, AOAC INTERNATIONAL, Book of Methods,[1] or in other recognized standard references, or is detailed in an approved new drug application and the referenced method is not modified, a statement indicating the method and reference will suffice). The suitability of all testing methods used shall be verified under actual conditions of use.

(3) A statement of the weight or measure of sample used for each test, where appropriate.

(4) A complete record of all data secured in the course of each test, including all graphs, charts, and spectra from laboratory instrumentation, properly identified to show the specific component, drug product container, closure, in-process material, or drug product, and lot tested.

---

[1]Copies may be obtained from: AOAC INTERNATIONAL, 481 North Frederick Ave., suite 500, Gaithersburg, MD 20877

(5) A record of all calculations performed in connection with the test, including units of measure, conversion factors, and equivalency factors.

(6) A statement of the results of tests and how the results compare with established standards of identity, strength, quality, and purity for the component, drug productcontainer, closure, in-process material, or drug product tested.

(7) The initials or signature of the person who performs each test and the date(s) the tests were performed.

(8) The initials or signature of a second person showing that the original records have been reviewed for accuracy, completeness, and compliance with established standards.

(b) Complete records shall be maintained of any modification of an established method employed in testing. Such records shall include the reason for the modification and data to verify that the modification produced results that are at least as accurate and reliable for the material being tested as the established method.

(c) Complete records shall be maintained of any testing and standardization of laboratory reference standards, reagents, and standard solutions.

(d) Complete records shall be maintained of the periodic calibration of laboratory instruments, apparatus, gauges, and recording devices required by §211.160(b)(4).

(e) Complete records shall be maintained of all stability testing performed in accordance with §211.166.

[43 FR 45077, Sept. 29, 1978, as amended at 55 FR 11577, Mar. 29, 1990; 65 FR 18889, Apr. 10, 2000; 70 FR 40880, July 15, 2005; 70 FR 67651, Nov. 8, 2005]

§211.196   Distribution records.

Distribution records shall contain the name and strength of the product and description of the dosage form, name and address of the consignee, date and quantity shipped, and lot or control number of the drug product. For compressed medical gas products, distribution records are not required to contain lot or control numbers.

(Approved by the Office of Management and Budget under control number 0910-0139) [49 FR 9865, Mar. 16, 1984]

§211.198   Complaint files.

(a) Written procedures describing the handling of all written and oral complaints regarding a drug product shall be established and followed. Such procedures shall include provisions for review by the quality control unit, of any complaint involving the possible failure of a drug product to meet any of its specifications and, for such drug products, a determination as to the need for an investigation in accordance with §211.192. Such procedures shall include provisions for review to determine whether the complaint represents a serious and unexpected adverse drug experience which is required to be reported to the Food and Drug Administration in accordance with §§310.305 and 514.80 of this chapter.

(b) A written record of each complaint shall be maintained in a file designated for drug product complaints. The file regarding such drug product complaints shall be maintained at the establishment where the drug product involved was manufactured, processed, or packed, or such file may be maintained at another facility if the written records in such files are readily available for inspection at that other facility. Written records involving a drug product shall be maintained until at least 1 year after the expiration date of the drug product, or 1 year after the date that the complaint was received, whichever is longer. In the case of certain OTC drug products lacking expiration dating because they meet the criteria for exemption under §211.137, such written records shall be maintained for 3 years after distribution of the drug product.

(1) The written record shall include the following information, where known: the name and strength of the drug product, lot number, name of complainant, nature of complaint, and reply to complainant.

(2) Where an investigation under §211.192 is conducted, the written record shall include the findings of the investigation and follow up. The record or copy of the record of the investigation shall be maintained at the establishment where the investigation occurred in accordance with §211.180(c).

(3) Where an investigation under §211.192 is not conducted, the written record shall include the reason that an investigation was found not to be necessary and the name of the responsible person making such a determination.

[43 FR 45077, Sept. 29, 1978, as amended at 51 FR 24479, July 3, 1986; 68 FR 15364, Mar. 31,2003]

Subpart K--Returned and Salvaged Drug Products

§211.204   Returned drug products.

Returned drug products shall be identified as such and held. If the conditions under which returned drug products have been held, stored, or shipped before or during their return, or if the condition of the drug product, its container, carton, or labeling, as a result of storage or shipping, casts doubt on the safety, identity, strength, quality or purity of the drug product, the returned drug product shall be destroyed unless examination, testing, or other investigations prove the drug product meets appropriate standards of safety, identity, strength, quality, or purity. A drug product may be reprocessed provided the subsequent drug product meets appropriate standards, specifications, and characteristics. Records of returned drug products shall be maintained and shall include the name and label potency of the drug product dosage form, lot number (or control number or batch number), reason for the return, quantity returned, date of disposition, and ultimate disposition of the returned drug product. If the reason for a drug product being returned implicates associated batches, an appropriate investigation shall be conducted in accordance with the requirements of §211.192. Procedures for the holding, testing, and reprocessing of returned drug products shall be in writing and shall be followed.

§211.208   Drug product salvaging.

Drug products that have been subjected to improper storage conditions including extremes in temperature, humidity, smoke, fumes, pressure, age, or radiation due to natural disasters, fires, accidents, or equipment failures shall not be salvaged and returned to the marketplace. Whenever there is a question whether drug products have been subjected to such conditions, salvaging operations may be conducted only if there is (a) evidence from laboratory tests and assays (including animal feeding studies where applicable) that the drug products meet all applicable standards of identity, strength, quality, and purity and (b) evidence from inspection of the premises that the drug products and their associated packaging were not subjected to improper storage conditions as a result of the disaster or accident. Organoleptic examinations shall be acceptable only as supplemental evidence that the drug products meet appropriate standards of identity, strength, quality, and purity. Records including name, lot number, and disposition shall be maintained for drug products subject to this section.

Notes

The Code of Federal Regulations
Title 21 – Food and Drugs

Part 600
BIOLOGICAL PRODUCTS: GENERAL

Printed by GMP Publications, Inc.
Tel: 866-544-9007 or 856-810-7331
Fax: 866-544-9002
http://www.gmppublications.com
sales@gmppublications.com

PART 600--BIOLOGICAL PRODUCTS: GENERAL

Authority: 21 U.S.C. 321, 351, 352, 353, 355, 356c, 356e, 360, 360i, 371, 374, 379k-1; 42 U.S.C. 216, 262, 263, 263a, 264

Cross References: For U.S. Customs Service regulations relating to viruses, serums, and toxins, see 19 CFR 12.21-12.23. For U.S. Postal Service regulations relating to the admissibility to the United States mails see parts 124 and 125 of the Domestic Mail Manual, that is incorporated by reference in 39 CFR part 111.

Subpart A--General Provisions

§600.2 Mailing addresses.

(a) *Licensed biological products regulated by the Center for Biologics Evaluation and Research (CBER).* Unless otherwise stated in paragraph (c) of this section, or as otherwise prescribed by FDA regulation, all submissions to CBER referenced in parts 600 through 680 of this chapter, as applicable, must be sent to: Food and Drug Administration, Center for Biologics Evaluation and Research, Document Control Center, 10903 New Hampshire Ave., Bldg. 71, Rm. G112, Silver Spring, MD 20993-0002. Examples of such submissions include: Biologics license applications (BLAs) and their amendments and supplements, biological product deviation reports, fatality reports, and other correspondence. Biological products samples must not be sent to this address but must be sent to the address in paragraph (c) of this section

(b) *Licensed biological products regulated by the Center for Drug Evaluation and Research (CDER).* Unless otherwise stated in paragraphs (b)(1), (b)(2), or (c) of this section, or as otherwise prescribed by FDA regulation, all submissions to CDER referenced in parts 600, 601, and 610 of this chapter, as applicable, must be sent to: CDER Central Document Room, Center for Drug Evaluation and Research, Food and Drug Administration, 5901B Ammendale Rd., Beltsville, MD 20705. Examples of such submissions include: BLAs and their amendments and supplements, and other correspondence.

(1) *Biological Product Deviation Reporting (CDER).* All biological product deviation reports required under §600.14 must be sent to: Division of Compliance Risk Management and Surveillance, Office of Compliance, Center for Drug Evaluation and Research, Food and Drug Administration, 10903 New Hampshire Ave., Silver Spring, MD 20993-0002.

(2) *Postmarketing Adverse Experience Reporting (CDER).* All advertising and promotional labeling supplements required under §601.12(f) of this chapter must be sent to: Division of Drug Marketing, Advertising and Communication, Center for Drug Evaluation and Research, Food and Drug Administration, 5901-B Ammendale Rd., Beltsville, MD 20705-1266

(3) *Advertising and Promotional Labeling (CDER).* All advertising and promotional labeling supplements required under §601.12(f) of this chapter must be sent to: Division of Drug Marketing, Advertising and Communication, Center for Drug Evaluation and Research, Food and Drug Administration, 5901-B Ammendale Rd., Beltsville, MD 20705-1266.

(c) *Samples and Protocols for licensed biological products regulated by CBER or CDER.* (1) Biological product samples and/or protocols, other than radioactive biological product samples and protocols, required under §§600.13, 600.22, 601.15, 610.2, 660.6, 660.36, or 660.46 of this chapter must be sent by courier service to: Food and Drug Administration, Center for Biologics Evaluation and Research, ATTN: Sample Custodian, 10903 New Hampshire Ave., Bldg. 75, Rm. G707, Silver Spring, MD 20993-0002. The protocol(s) may be placed in the box used to ship the samples to CBER. A cover letter should not be included when submitting the protocol with the sample unless it contains pertinent information affecting the release of the lot.

(2) Radioactive biological products required under §610.2 of this chapter must be sent by courier service to: Food and Drug Administration, Center for Biologics Evaluation and Research, ATTN: Sample Custodian, c/o White Oak Radiation Safety Program, 10903 New Hampshire Ave., Bldg. 52-72, Rm. G406A, Silver Spring, MD 20993-0002.

(d) Address information for submissions to CBER and CDER other than those listed in parts 600 through 680 of this chapter are included directly in the applicable regulations.

(e) Obtain updated mailing address information for biological products regulated by CBER at http://www.fda.gov/BiologicsBloodVaccines/default.htm, or for biological products regulated by CDER at http://www.fda.gov/Drugs/default.htm.

[70 FR 14981, Mar. 24, 2005, as amended at 74 FR 13114, Mar. 26, 2009; 78 FR 19585, Apr. 2, 2013; 80 FR 18091, Apr. 3, 2015; 79 FR 33090, June 10, 2014]

§600.3   Definitions.

As used in this subchapter:

(a) *Act* means the Public Health Service Act (58 Stat. 682), approved July 1, 1944.

(b) *Secretary* means the Secretary of Health and Human Services and any other officer or employee of the Department of Health and Human Services to whom the authority involved has been delegated.

(c) *Commissioner of Food and Drugs* means the Commissioner of the Food and Drug Administration.

(d) *Center for Biologics Evaluation and Research* means Center for Biologics Evaluation and Research of the Food and Drug Administration.

(e) *State* means a State or the District of Columbia, Puerto Rico, or the Virgin Islands.

(f) *Possession* includes among other possessions, Puerto Rico and the Virgin Islands.

(g) *Products* includes biological products and trivalent organic arsenicals.

(h) *Biological product* means a virus, therapeutic serum, toxin, antitoxin, vaccine, blood, blood component or derivative, allergenic product, protein, or analogous product, or arsphenamine or derivative of arsphenamine (or any other trivalent organic arsenic compound), applicable to the prevention, treatment, or cure of a disease or condition of human beings.

(1) A virus is interpreted to be a product containing the minute living cause of an infectious disease and includes but is not limited to filterable viruses, bacteria, rickettsia, fungi, and protozoa.

(2) A therapeutic serum is a product obtained from blood by removing the clot or clot components and the blood cells.

(3) A toxin is a product containing a soluble substance poisonous to laboratory animals or to man in doses of 1 milliliter or less (or equivalent in weight) of the product, and having the property, following the injection of non-fatal doses into an animal, of causing to be produced therein another soluble substance which specifically neutralizes the poisonous substance and which is demonstrable in the serum of the animal thus immunized.

(4) An antitoxin is a product containing the soluble substance in serum or other body fluid of an immunized animal which specifically neutralizes the toxin against which the animal is immune.

(5) A product is analogous:

(i) To a virus if prepared from or with a virus or agent actually or potentially infectious, without regard to the degree of virulence or toxicogenicity of the specific strain used.

(ii) To a therapeutic serum, if composed of whole blood or plasma or containing some organic constituent or product other than a hormone or an amino acid, derived from whole blood, plasma, or serum.

(iii) To a toxin or antitoxin, if intended, irrespective of its source of origin, to be applicable to the prevention, treatment, or cure of disease or injuries of man through a specific immune process.

(6) A protein is any alpha amino acid polymer with a specific, defined sequence that is greater than 40 amino acids in size. When two or more amino acid chains in an amino acid polymer are associated with each other in a manner that occurs in nature, the size of the amino acid polymer for purposes of this paragraph (h)(6) will be based on the total number of amino acids in those chains, and will not be limited to the number of amino acids in a contiguous sequence.

(i) *Trivalent organic arsenicals* means arsphenamine and its derivatives (or any other trivalent organic arsenic compound) applicable to the prevention, treatment, or cure of diseases or injuries of man.

(j) A product is deemed *applicable to the prevention, treatment, or cure of diseases or injuries of man* irrespective of the mode of administration or application recommended, including use when intended through administration or application to a person as an aid in diagnosis, or in evaluating the degree of susceptibility or immunity possessed by a person, and including also any other use for purposes of diagnosis if the diagnostic substance so used is prepared from or with the aid of a biological product.

(k) *Proper name*, as applied to a product, means the name designated in the license for use upon each package of the product.

(l) *Dating period* means the period beyond which the product cannot be expected beyond reasonable doubt to yield its specific results.

(m) *Expiration date* means the calendar month and year, and where applicable, the day and hour, that the dating period ends.

(n) The word *standards* means specifications and procedures applicable to an establishment or to the manufacture or release of products, which are prescribed in this subchapter or established in the biologics license application designed to insure the continued safety, purity, and potency of such products.

(o) The word *continued* as applied to the safety, purity and potency of products is interpreted to apply to the dating period.

(p) The word *safety* means the relative freedom from harmful effect to persons affected, directly or indirectly, by a product when prudently administered, taking into consideration the character of the product in relation to the condition of the recipient at the time.

(q) The word *sterility* is interpreted to mean freedom from viable contaminating microorganisms, as determined by the tests conducted under in §610.12 of this chapter.

(r) *Purity* means relative freedom from extraneous matter in the finished product, whether or not harmful to the recipient or deleterious to the product. *Purity* includes but is not limited to relative freedom from residual moisture or other volatile substances and pyrogenic substances.

(s) The word *potency* is interpreted to mean the specific ability or capacity of the product, as indicated by appropriate laboratory tests or by adequately controlled clinical data obtained through the administration of the product in the manner intended, to effect a given result.

(t) *Manufacturer* means any legal person or entity engaged in the manufacture of a product subject to license under the act; "Manufacturer" also includes any legal person or entity who is an applicant for a license where the applicant assumes responsibility for compliance with the applicable product and establishment standards.

(u) *Manufacture* means all steps in propagation or manufacture and preparation of products and includes but is not limited to filling, testing, labeling, packaging, and storage by the manufacturer.

(v) *Location* includes all buildings, appurtenances, equipment and animals used, and personnel engaged by a manufacturer within a particular area designated by an address adequate for identification.

(w) *Establishment* has the same meaning as "facility" in section 351 of the Public Health Service Act and includes all locations.

(x) *Lot* means that quantity of uniform material identified by the manufacturer as having been thoroughly mixed in a single vessel.

(y) *A filling* refers to a group of final containers identical in all respects, which have been filled with the same product from the same bulk lot without any change that will affect the integrity of the filling assembly.

(z) *Process* refers to a manufacturing step that is performed on the product itself which may affect its safety, purity or potency, in contrast to such manufacturing steps which do not affect intrinsically the safety, purity or potency of the product.

(aa) *Selling agent* or *distributor* means any person engaged in the unrestricted distribution, other than by sale at retail, of products subject to license.

(bb) *Container* (referred to also as "final container") is the immediate unit, bottle, vial, ampule, tube, or other receptacle containing the product as distributed for sale, barter, or exchange.

(cc) *Package* means the immediate carton, receptacle, or wrapper, including all labeling matter therein and thereon, and the contents of the one or more enclosed containers. If no package, as defined in the preceding sentence, is used, the container shall be deemed to be the package.

(dd) *Label* means any written, printed, or graphic matter on the container or package or any such matter clearly visible through the immediate carton, receptacle, or wrapper.

(ee) *Radioactive biological product* means a biological product which is labeled with a radionuclide or intended solely to be labeled with a radionuclide.

(ff) *Amendment* is the submission of information to a pending license application or supplement, to revise or modify the application as originally submitted.

(gg) *Supplement* is a request to approve a change in an approved license application.

(hh) *Distributed* means the biological product has left the control of the licensed manufacturer.

(ii) *Control* means having responsibility for maintaining the continued safety, purity, and potency of the product and for compliance with applicable product and establishment standards, and for compliance with current good manufacturing practices.

(jj) *Assess the effects of the change*, as used in § 601.12 of this chapter, means to evaluate the effects of a manufacturing change on the identity, strength, quality, purity, and potency of a product as these factors may relate to the safety or effectiveness of the product.

(kk) *Specification*, as used in §601.12 of this chapter, means the quality standard (i.e., tests, analytical procedures, and acceptance criteria) provided in an approved application to confirm the quality of products, intermediates, raw materials, reagents, components, in-process materials, container closure systems, and other materials used in the production of a product. For the purpose of this definition, *acceptance criteria* means numerical limits, ranges, or other criteria for the tests described.

(ll) *Complete response letter* means a written communication to an applicant from FDA usually describing all of the deficiencies that the agency has identified in a biologics license application or supplement that must be satisfactorily addressed before it can be approved.

(mm) *Resubmission* means a submission by the biologics license applicant or supplement applicant of all materials needed to fully address all deficiencies identified in the complete response letter. A biologics license application or supplement for which FDA issued a complete response letter, but which was withdrawn before approval and later submitted again, is not a resubmission.

[38 FR 32048, Nov. 20, 1973, as amended at 40 FR 31313, July 25, 1975; 55 FR 11014, Mar. 26, 1990; 61 FR 24232, May 14, 1996; 62 FR 39901, July 24, 1997; 64 FR 56449, Oct. 20, 1999; 65 FR 66634, Nov. 7, 2000; 69 FR 18766, Apr. 8, 2004; 70 FR 14982, Mar. 24, 2005; 73 FR 39610, July 10, 2008; 77 FR 26174, May 3, 2012; 85 FR 10063, Mar. 23, 2020]

Subpart B--Establishment Standards

§600.10 Personnel.

(a) [Reserved]

(b) *Personnel.* Personnel shall have capabilities commensurate with their assigned functions, a thorough understanding of the manufacturing operations which they perform, the necessary training and experience relating to individual products, and adequate information concerning the application of the pertinent provisions of this subchapter to their respective functions. Personnel shall include such professionally trained persons as are necessary to insure the competent performance of all manufacturing processes.

(c) *Restrictions on personnel—*(1) *Specific duties.* Persons whose presence can affect adversely the safety and purity of a product shall be excluded from the room where the manufacture of a product is in progress.

(2) *Sterile operations.* Personnel performing sterile operations shall wear clean or sterilized protective clothing and devices to the extent necessary to protect the product from contamination.

(3) *Pathogenic viruses and spore-bearing organisms.* Persons working with viruses pathogenic for man or with spore-forming microorganisms, and persons engaged in the care of animals or animal quarters, shall be excluded from areas where other products are manufactured, or such persons shall change outer clothing, including shoes, or wear protective covering prior to entering such areas.

(4) *Live vaccine work areas.* Persons may not enter a live vaccine processing area after having worked with

other infectious agents in any other laboratory during the same working day. Only persons actually concerned with propagation of the culture, production of the vaccine, and unit maintenance, shall be allowed in live vaccine processing areas when active work is in progress. Casual visitors shall be excluded from such units at all times and all others having business in such areas shall be admitted only under supervision. Street clothing, including shoes, shall be replaced or covered by suitable laboratory clothing before entering a live vaccine processing unit. Persons caring for animals used in the manufacture of live vaccines shall be excluded from other animal quarters and from contact with other animals during the same working day.

[38 FR 32048, Nov. 20, 1973, as amended at 49 FR 23833, June 8, 1984; 55 FR 11014, Mar. 26, 1990; 62 FR 53538, Oct. 15, 1997; 68 FR 75119, Dec. 30, 2003]

§600.11   Physical establishment, equipment, animals, and care.

(a) *Work areas.* All rooms and work areas where products are manufactured or stored shall be kept orderly, clean, and free of dirt, dust, vermin and objects not required for manufacturing. Precautions shall be taken to avoid clogging and back-siphonage of drainage systems. Precautions shall be taken to exclude extraneous infectious agents from manufacturing areas. Work rooms shall be well lighted and ventilated. The ventilation system shall be arranged so as to prevent the dissemination of microorganisms from one manufacturing area to another and to avoid other conditions unfavorable to the safety of the product. Filling rooms, and other rooms where open, sterile operations are conducted, shall be adequate to meet manufacturing needs and such rooms shall be constructed and equipped to permit thorough cleaning and to keep air-borne contaminants at a minimum. If such rooms are used for other purposes, they shall be cleaned and prepared prior to use for sterile operations. Refrigerators, incubators and warm rooms shall be maintained at temperatures within applicable ranges and shall be free of extraneous material which might affect the safety of the product.

(b) *Equipment.* Apparatus for sterilizing equipment and the method of operation shall be such as to insure the destruction of contaminating microorganisms. The effectiveness of the sterilization procedure shall be no less than that achieved by an attained temperature of 121.5°C maintained for 20 minutes by saturated steam or by an attained temperature of 170°C maintained for 2 hours with dry heat. Processing and storage containers, filters, filling apparatus, and other pieces of apparatus and accessory equipment, including pipes and tubing, shall be designed and constructed to permit thorough cleaning and, where possible, inspection for cleanliness. All surfaces that come in contact with products shall be clean and free of surface solids, leachable contaminants, and other materials that will hasten the deterioration of the product or otherwise render it less suitable for the intended use. For products for which sterility is a factor, equipment shall be sterile, unless sterility of the product is assured by subsequent procedures.

(c) *Laboratory and bleeding rooms.* Rooms used for the processing of products, including bleeding rooms, shall be effectively fly-proofed and kept free of flies and vermin. Such rooms shall be so constructed as to insure freedom from dust, smoke and other deleterious substances and to permit thorough cleaning and disinfection. Rooms for animal injection and bleeding, and rooms for smallpox vaccine animals, shall be disinfected and be provided with the necessary water, electrical and other services.

(d) *Animal quarters and stables.* Animal quarters, stables and food storage areas shall be of appropriate construction, fly-proofed, adequately lighted and ventilated, and maintained in a clean, vermin-free and sanitary condition. No manure or refuse shall be stored as to permit the breeding of flies on the premises, nor shall the establishment be located in close proximity to off-property manure or refuse storage capable of engendering fly breeding.

(e) *Restrictions on building and equipment use*—(1) *Work of a diagnostic nature.* Laboratory procedures of a clinical diagnostic nature involving materials that may be contaminated, shall not be performed in space used for the manufacture of products except that manufacturing space which is used only occasionally may be used for diagnostic work provided spore-forming pathogenic microorganisms are not involved and provided the space is thoroughly cleaned and disinfected before the manufacture of products is resumed.

(2) *Spore-forming organisms for supplemental sterilization procedure control test.* Spore-forming organisms used as an additional control in sterilization procedures may be introduced into areas used for the manufacture of products, only for the purposes of the test and only immediately before use for such purposes: *Provided,* That (i) the organism is not pathogenic for man or animals and does not produce pyrogens or toxins, (ii) the culture is demonstrated to be pure, (iii) transfer of test cultures to culture media shall be limited to the sterility test area or areas designated for work with spore-forming organisms, (iv) each culture be labeled with the name of the microorganism and the statement "Caution: microbial spores. See directions for storage, use and disposition.", and (v) the container of each culture is designed to withstand handling without breaking.

(3) *Work with spore-forming microorganisms.* (i) Manufacturing processes using spore-forming microorganisms conducted in a multiproduct manufacturing site must be performed under appropriate controls to prevent contamination of other products and areas within the site. Prevention of spore contamination can be achieved by using a separate dedicated building or by using process containment if manufacturing is conducted in a multiproduct manufacturing building. All product and personnel movement between the area where the spore-forming microorganisms are manufactured and other manufacturing areas must be conducted under conditions that will prevent the introduction of spores into other areas of the facility.

(ii) If process containment is employed in a multiproduct manufacturing area, procedures must be in place to demonstrate adequate removal of the spore-forming microorganism(s) from the manufacturing area for subsequent manufacture of other products. These procedures must provide for adequate removal or decontamination of the spore-forming microorganisms on and within manufacturing equipment, facilities, and ancillary room items as well as the removal of disposable or product dedicated items from the manufacturing area. Environmental monitoring specific for the spore-forming microorganism(s) must be conducted in adjacent areas during manufacturing operations and in the manufacturing area after completion of cleaning and decontamination.

(4) *Live vaccine processing.* Live vaccine processing must be performed under appropriate controls to prevent cross contamination of other products and other manufacturing areas within the building. Appropriate controls must include, at a minimum:

(i)(A) Using a dedicated manufacturing area that is either in a separate building, in a separate wing of a building, or in quarters at the blind end of a corridor and includes adequate space and equipment for all processing steps up to, but not including, filling into final containers; and

(B) Not conducting test procedures that potentially involve the presence of microorganisms other than the vaccine strains or the use of tissue culture cell lines other than primary cultures in space used for processing live vaccine; or

(ii) If manufacturing is conducted in a multiproduct manufacturing building or area, using procedural controls, and where necessary, process containment. Process containment is deemed to be necessary unless procedural controls are sufficient to prevent cross contamination of other products and other manufacturing areas within the building. Process containment is a system designed to mechanically isolate equipment or an area that involves manufacturing using live vaccine organisms. All product, equipment, and personnel movement between distinct live vaccine processing areas and between live vaccine processing areas and other manufacturing areas, up to, but not including, filling in final containers, must be conducted under conditions that will prevent cross contamination of other products and manufacturing areas within the building, including the introduction of live vaccine organisms into other areas. In addition, written procedures and effective processes must be in place to adequately remove or decontaminate live vaccine organisms from the manufacturing area and equipment for subsequent manufacture of other products. Written procedures must be in place for verification that processes to remove or decontaminate live vaccine organisms have been followed.

(5) *Equipment and supplies—contamination.* Equipment and supplies used in work on or otherwise exposed to any pathogenic or potentially pathogenic agent shall be kept separated from equipment and supplies used in the manufacture of products to the extent necessary to prevent cross-contamination.

(f) *Animals used in manufacture*—(1) *Care of animals used in manufacturing.* Caretakers and attendants for animals used for the manufacture of products shall be sufficient in number and have adequate experience to insure adequate care. Animal quarters and cages shall be kept in sanitary condition. Animals on production shall be inspected daily to observe response to production procedures. Animals that become ill for reasons not related to production shall be isolated from other animals and shall not be used for production until recovery is complete. Competent veterinary care shall be provided as needed.

(2) *Quarantine of animals*—(i) *General.* No animal shall be used in processing unless kept under competent daily inspection and preliminary quarantine for a period of at least 7 days before use, or as otherwise provided in this subchapter. Only healthy animals free from detectable communicable diseases shall be used. Animals must remain in overt good health throughout the quarantine

periods and particular care shall be taken during the quarantine periods to reject animals of the equine genus which may be infected with glanders and animals which may be infected with tuberculosis.

(ii) *Quarantine of monkeys*. In addition to observing the pertinent general quarantine requirements, monkeys used as a source of tissue in the manufacture of vaccine shall be maintained in quarantine for at least 6 weeks prior to use, except when otherwise provided in this part. Only monkeys that have reacted negatively to tuberculin at the start of the quarantine period and again within 2 weeks prior to use shall be used in the manufacture of vaccine. Due precaution shall be taken to prevent cross-infection from any infected or potentially infected monkeys on the premises. Monkeys to be used in the manufacture of a live vaccine shall be maintained throughout the quarantine period in cages closed on all sides with solid materials except the front which shall be screened, with no more than two monkeys housed in one cage. Cage mates shall not be interchanged.

(3) *Immunization against tetanus*. Horses and other animals susceptible to tetanus, that are used in the processing steps of the manufacture of biological products, shall be treated adequately to maintain immunity to tetanus.

(4) *Immunization and bleeding of animals used as a source of products*. Toxins or other nonviable antigens administered in the immunization of animals used in the manufacture of products shall be sterile. Viable antigens, when so used, shall be free of contaminants, as determined by appropriate tests prior to use. Injections shall not be made into horses within 6 inches of bleeding site. Horses shall not be bled for manufacturing purposes while showing persistent general reaction or local reaction near the site of bleeding. Blood shall not be used if it was drawn within 5 days of injecting the animals with viable microorganisms. Animals shall not be bled for manufacturing purposes when they have an intercurrent disease. Blood intended for use as a source of a biological product shall be collected in

clean, sterile vessels. When the product is intended for use by injection, such vessels shall also be pyrogen-free.

(5) [Reserved]

(6) *Reporting of certain diseases.* In cases of actual or suspected infection with foot and mouth disease, glanders, tetanus, anthrax, gas gangrene, equine infectious anemia; equine encephalomyelitis, or any of the pock diseases among animals intended for use or used in the manufacture of products, the manufacturer shall immediately notify the Director, Center for Biologics Evaluation and Research or the Director, Center for Drug Evaluation and Research (see mailing addresses in §600.2(a) or (b)).

(7) *Monkeys used previously for experimental or test purposes.* Monkeys that have been used previously for experimental or test purposes with live microbiological agents shall not be used as a source of kidney tissue for the manufacture of vaccine. Except as provided otherwise in this subchapter, monkeys that have been used previously for other experimental or test purposes may be used as a source of kidney tissue upon their return to a normal condition, provided all quarantine requirements have been met.

(8) *Necropsy examination of monkeys.* Each monkey used in the manufacture of vaccine shall be examined at necropsy under the direction of a qualified pathologist, physician, or veterinarian having experience with diseases of monkeys, for evidence of ill health, particularly for (i) evidence of tuberculosis, (ii) presence of herpes-like lesions, including eruptions or plaques on or around the lips, in the buccal cavity or on the gums, and (iii) signs of conjunctivitis. If there are any such signs or other significant gross pathological lesions, the tissue shall not be used in the manufacture of vaccine.

(g) *Filling procedures.* Filling procedures shall be such as will not affect adversely the safety, purity or potency of the product.

(h) *Containers and closures.* All final containers and closures shall be made of material that will not hasten the deterioration of the product or otherwise render it less suitable for the intended use. All final containers and closures shall be clean and free of surface solids, leachable contaminants and other materials that will hasten the deterioration of the product or otherwise render it less suitable for the intended use. After filling, sealing shall be performed in a manner that will maintain the integrity of the product during the dating period. In addition, final containers and closures for products intended for use by injection shall be sterile and free from pyrogens. Except as otherwise provided in the regulations of this subchapter, final containers for products intended for use by injection shall be colorless and sufficiently transparent to permit visual examination of the contents under normal light. As soon as possible after filling final containers shall be labeled as prescribed in §610.60 *et seq.* of this chapter, except that final containers may be stored without such prescribed labeling provided they are stored in a sealed receptacle labeled both inside and outside with at least the name of the product, the lot number, and the filling identification.

[38 FR 32048, Nov. 20, 1973, as amended at 41 FR 10428, Mar. 11, 1976; 49 FR 23833, June 8, 1984; 55 FR 11013, Mar. 26, 1990; 68 FR 75119, Dec. 30, 2003; 70 FR 14982, Mar. 24, 2005; 72 FR 59003, Oct. 18, 2007; 80 FR 18092, Apr. 3, 2015]

§600.12   Records.

(a) *Maintenance of records.* Records shall be made, concurrently with the performance, of each step in the manufacture and distribution of products, in such a manner that at any time successive steps in the manufacture and distribution of any lot may be traced by an inspector. Such records shall be legible and indelible, shall identify the person immediately responsible, shall include dates of the various steps, and be as detailed as necessary for clear understanding of each step by one experienced in the manufacture of products.

(b) *Records retention*—(1) *General.* Records shall be retained for such interval beyond the expiration date as is necessary for the individual product, to permit the return of any clinical report of unfavorable reactions. The retention period shall be no less than five years after the records of manufacture have been completed or six months after the latest expiration date for the individual product, whichever represents a later date.

(2) *Records of recall.* Complete records shall be maintained pertaining to the recall from distribution of any product upon notification by the Director, Center for Biologics Evaluation and Research or the Director, Center for Drug Evaluation and Research to recall for failure to conform with the standards prescribed in the regulations of this subchapter, because of deterioration of the product or for any other factor by reason of which the distribution of the product would constitute a danger to health.

(3) *Suspension of requirement for retention.* The Director, Center for Biologics Evaluation and Research or the Director, Center for Drug Evaluation and Research may authorize the suspension of the requirement to retain records of a specific manufacturing step upon a showing that such records no longer have significance for the purposes for which they were made: Provided, That a summary of such records shall be retained.

(c) *Records of sterilization of equipment and supplies.* Records relating to the mode of sterilization, date, duration, temperature and other conditions relating to each sterilization of equipment and supplies used in the processing of products shall be made by means of automatic recording devices or by means of a system of recording which gives equivalent assurance of the accuracy and reliability of the record. Such records shall be maintained in a manner that permits an identification of the product with the particular manufacturing process to which the sterilization relates.

(d) *Animal necropsy records.* A necropsy record shall be kept on each animal from which a biological product has been obtained and which dies or is sacrificed while being so used.

(e) *Records in case of divided manufacturing responsibility.* If two or more establishments participate in the manufacture of a product, the records of each such establishment must show plainly the degree of its responsibility. In addition, each participating manufacturer shall furnish to the manufacturer who prepares the product in final form for sale, barter or exchange, a copy of all records relating to the manufacturing operations performed by such participating manufacturer insofar as they concern the safety, purity and potency of the lots of the product involved, and the manufacturer who prepares the product in final form shall retain a complete record of all the manufacturing operations relating to the product.

[38 FR 32048, Nov. 20, 1973, as amended at 49 FR 23833, June 8, 1984; 55 FR 11013, Mar. 26, 1990; 70 FR 14982, Mar. 24, 2005]

§600.13   Retention samples.

Manufacturers shall retain for a period of at least 6 months after the expiration date, unless a different time period is specified in additional standards, a quantity of representative material of each lot of each product, sufficient for examination and testing for safety and potency, except Whole Blood, Cryoprecipitated AHF, Platelets, Red Blood Cells, Plasma, and Source Plasma and Allergenic Products prepared to a physician's prescription. Samples so retained shall be selected at random from either final container material, or from bulk and final containers, provided they include at least one final container as a final package, or package-equivalent of such filling of each lot of the product as intended for distribution. Such sample material shall be stored at temperatures and under conditions which will maintain the identity and integrity of the product. Samples retained as required in this section shall be in addition to samples of specific products required to be submitted to the Center for Biologics Evaluation and Research or the Center for Drug Evaluation and Research (see mailing addresses in §600.2). Exceptions may be authorized by the Director, Center for Biologics Evaluation and Research or the Director, Center for Drug Evaluation and Research, when the lot yields relatively few final containers and when such lots are prepared by the same method in large number and in close succession.

[41 FR 10428, Mar. 11, 1976, as amended at 49 FR 23833, June 8, 1984; 50 FR 4133, Jan. 29, 1985; 55 FR 11013, Mar. 26, 1990; 70 FR 14982, Mar. 24, 2005]

§600.14   Reporting of biological product deviations by licensed manufacturers.

(a) *Who must report under this section?* (1) You, the manufacturer who holds the biological product license and who had control over the product when the deviation occurred, must report under this section. If you arrange for another person to perform a manufacturing, holding, or distribution step, while the product is in your control, that step is performed under your control. You must establish, maintain, and follow a procedure for receiving information from that person on all deviations, complaints, and adverse events concerning the affected product.

(2) Exceptions:

(i) Persons who manufacture only in vitro diagnostic products that are not subject to licensing under section 351 of the Public Health Service Act do not report biological product deviations for those products under this section but must report in accordance with part 803 of this chapter;

(ii) Persons who manufacture blood and blood components, including licensed manufacturers, unlicensed registered blood establishments, and transfusion services, do not report biological product deviations for those products under this section but must report under §606.171 of this chapter;

(iii) Persons who manufacture Source Plasma or any other blood component and use that Source Plasma or any other blood component in the further manufacture of another licensed biological product must report:

(A) Under §606.171 of this chapter, if a biological product deviation occurs during the manufacture of that Source Plasma or any other blood component; or

(B) Under this section, if a biological product deviation occurs after the manufacture of that Source Plasma or any other blood component, and during manufacture of the licensed biological product.

(b) *What do I report under this section?* You must report

any event, and information relevant to the event, associated with the manufacturing, to include testing, processing, packing, labeling, or storage, or with the holding or distribution, of a licensed biological product, if that event meets all the following criteria:

(1) Either:

(i) Represents a deviation from current good manufacturing practice, applicable regulations, applicable standards, or established specifications that may affect the safety, purity, or potency of that product; or

(ii) Represents an unexpected or unforeseeable event that may affect the safety, purity, or potency of that product; and

(2) Occurs in your facility or another facility under contract with you; and

(3) Involves a distributed biological product.

(c) *When do I report under this section?* You should report a biological product deviation as soon as possible but you must report at a date not to exceed 45-calendar days from the date you, your agent, or another person who performs a manufacturing, holding, or distribution step under your control, acquire information reasonably suggesting that a reportable event has occurred.

(d) *How do I report under this section?* You must report on Form FDA-3486.

(e) *Where do I report under this section?* (1) For biological products regulated by the Center for Biologics Evaluation and Research (CBER), send the completed Form FDA 3486 to the CBER Document Control Center (see mailing address in §600.2(a)), or submit electronically using CBER's electronic Web-based application.

(2) For biological products regulated by the Center for Drug Evaluation and Research (CDER), send the completed Form FDA-3486 to the Division of Compliance Risk Management and Surveillance (HFD-330) (see mailing addresses in §600.2). CDER does not currently accept electronic filings.

(3) If you make a paper filing, you should identify on the envelope that a biological product deviation report (BPDR) is enclosed.

(f) *How does this regulation affect other FDA regulations?* This part supplements and does not supersede other provisions of the regulations in this chapter. All biological product deviations, whether or not they are required to be reported under this section, should be investigated in accordance with the applicable provisions of parts 211 and 820 of this chapter.

[65 FR 66634, Nov. 7, 2000, as amended at 70 FR 14982, Mar. 24, 2005; 80 FR 18092, Apr. 3, 2015]]

§600.15 Temperatures during shipment.

The following products shall be maintained during shipment at the specified temperatures:

(a) Products.

Product	Temperature
Cryoprecipitated AHF	-18 °C or colder.
Measles and Rubella Virus Vaccine Live	10 °C or colder.
Measles Live and Smallpox Vaccine	Do.
Measles, Mumps, and Rubella Virus Vaccine Live.	Do.
Measles and Mumps Virus Vaccine Live	Do.
Measles Virus Vaccine Live	Do.
Mumps Virus Vaccine Live	Do.
Fresh Frozen Plasma	-18 °C or colder.
Liquid Plasma	1 to 10 °C.
Plasma	-18 °C or colder.
Platelet Rich Plasma	Between 1 and 10 °C if the label indicates storage between 1 and 6 °C, or all reasonable methods to maintain the temperature as close as possible to a range between 20 and 24 °C, if the label indicates storage between 20 and 24 °C.
Platelets	Between 1 and 10 °C if the label indicates storage between 1 and 6 °C, or all reasonable methods to the temperature as close as possible to a range between 20 to 24 °C, if the label indicates storage between 20 and 24 °C.
Poliovirus Vaccine Live Oral Trivalent	0 °C or colder.
Poliovirus Vaccine Live Oral Type I	Do.
Poliovirus Vaccine Live Oral Type II	Do.
Poliovirus Vaccine Live Oral Type III	Do.
Red Blood Cells (liquid product)	Between 1 and 10 °C.
Red Blood Cells Frozen	-65 °C or colder.
Rubella and Mumps Virus Vaccine Live	10 °C or colder.
Rubella Virus Vaccine Live	Do.
Smallpox Vaccine (Liquid Product)	0 °C or colder.
Source Plasma	-5 °C or colder.
Source Plasma Liquid	10 °C or colder.

| Whole Blood | Blood that is transported from the collecting facility to the processing facility shall be transported in an environment capable of continuously cooling the blood toward a temperature range of 1 to 10 °C, or at a temperature as close as possible to 20 to 24 °C for a period not to exceed 6 hours. Blood transported from the storage facility shall be placed in an appropriate environment to maintain a temperature range between 1 to 10 °C during shipment. |
| Yellow Fever Vaccine | 0 °C or colder. |

(b) *Exemptions*. Exemptions or modifications shall be made only upon written approval, in the form of a supplement to the biologics license application, approved by the Director, Center for Biologics Evaluation and Research.

[39 FR 39872, Nov. 12, 1974, as amended at 49 FR 23833, June 8, 1984; 50 FR 4133, Jan. 29, 1985; 50 FR 9000, Mar. 6, 1985; 55 FR 11013, Mar. 26, 1990; 59 FR 49351, Sept. 28, 1994; 64 FR 56449, Oct. 20, 1999]

Subpart C--Establishment Inspection

§600.20   Inspectors.

Inspections shall be made by an officer of the Food and Drug Administration having special knowledge of the methods used in the manufacture and control of products and designated for such purposes by the Commissioner of Food and Drugs, or by any officer, agent, or employee of the Department of Health and Human Services specifically designated for such purpose by the Secretary.

[38 FR 32048, Nov. 20, 1973]

§600.21   Time of inspection.

The inspection of an establishment for which a biologics license application is pending need not be made until the establishment is in operation and is manufacturing the complete product for which a biologics license is desired.

[38 FR 32048, Nov. 20, 1973, as amended at 48 FR 26314, June 7, 1983; 64 FR 56449, Oct. 20, 1999; 84 FR 12508, Apr. 2, 2019]

§600.22 [Removed and Reserved]

Subpart D--Reporting of Adverse Experiences
Source: 59 FR 54042, Oct. 27, 1994, unless otherwise noted.

§600.80 Postmarketing reporting of adverse experiences.

(a) *Definitions*. The following definitions of terms apply to this section:

Adverse experience. Any adverse event associated with the use of a biological product in humans, whether or not considered product related, including the following: An adverse event occurring in the course of the use of a biological product in professional practice; an adverse event occurring from overdose of the product whether accidental or intentional; an adverse event occurring from abuse of the product; an adverse event occurring from withdrawal of the product; and any failure of expected pharmacological action.

Blood Component. As defined in §606.3(c) of this chapter.

Disability. A substantial disruption of a person's ability to conduct normal life functions.

Individual case safety report (ICSR). A description of an adverse experience related to an individual patient or subject.

ICSR attachments. Documents related to the adverse experience described in an ICSR, such as medical records, hospital discharge summaries, or other documentation.

Life-threatening adverse experience. Any adverse experience that places the patient, in the view of the initial reporter, at immediate risk of death from the adverse experience as it occurred, i.e., it does not include an adverse experience that, had it occurred in a more severe form, might have caused death.

Serious adverse experience. Any adverse experience occurring at any dose that results in any of the following outcomes: Death, a life-threatening adverse experience, inpatient hospitalization or prolongation of existing hospitalization, a persistent or significant disability/incapacity, or a congenital anomaly/birth defect. Important medical events that may not result in death, be life-threatening, or require hospitalization may be considered a serious adverse experience when, based upon appropriatemedical judgment, they may jeopardize the patient orsubject and may require medical or surgical intervention to prevent one of the outcomes listed in this definition. Examples of such medical events include allergic bronchospasm requiring intensive treatment in an emergency room or at home, blood dyscrasias or convulsions that do not result in inpatient hospitalization, or the development of drug dependency or drug abuse.

Unexpected adverse experience: Any adverse experience that is not listed in the current labeling for the biological product. This includes events that may be symptomatically and pathophysiologically related to an event listed in the labeling, but differ from the event because of greater severity or specificity. For example, under this definition, hepatic necrosis would be unexpected (by virtue of greater severity) if the labeling only referred to elevated hepatic enzymes or hepatitis. Similarly, cerebral thromboembolism and cerebral vasculitis would be unexpected (by virtue of greater specificity) if the labeling only listed cerebral vascular accidents. "Unexpected," as used in this definition, refers to an adverse experience that has not been previously observed (i.e., included in the labeling) rather than from the perspective of such experience not being anticipated from the pharmacological properties of the pharmaceutical product.

(b) *Review of adverse experiences*. Any person having a biologics license under §601.20 of this chapter must promptly review all adverse experience information pertaining to its product obtained or otherwise received by the applicant from any source, foreign or domestic, including information derived from commercial marketing experience, postmarketing clinical investigations, postmarketing epidemiological/surveillance studies, reports in the scientific literature, and unpublished scientific papers.

Applicants are not required to resubmit to FDA adverse product experience reports forwarded to the applicant by FDA; applicants, however, must submit all followup information on such reports to FDA. Any person subject to the reporting requirements under paragraph (c) of this section must also develop written procedures for the surveillance, receipt, evaluation, and reporting of postmarketing adverse experiences to FDA.

(c) *Reporting requirements.* The applicant must submit to FDA postmarketing 15-day Alert reports and periodic safety reports pertaining to its biological product as described in this section. These reports must be submitted to the Agency in electronic format as described in paragraph (h)(1) of this section, except as provided in paragraph (h)(2) of this section.

(1)(i) Postmarketing 15-day "Alert reports". The applicant must report each adverse experience that is both serious and unexpected, whether foreign or domestic, as soon as possible but no later than 15 calendar days from initial receipt of the information by the applicant.

(ii) *Postmarketing 15-day "Alert reports"*—followup. The applicant must promptly investigate all adverse experiences that are the subject of these postmarketing 15-day Alert reports and must submit followup reports within 15 calendar days of receipt of new information or as requested by FDA. If additional information is not obtainable, records should be maintained of the unsuccessful steps taken to seek additional information.

(iii) *Submission of reports.* The requirements of paragraphs (c)(1)(i) and (c)(1)(ii) of this section, concerning the submission of postmarketing 15-day Alert reports, also apply to any person whose name appears on the label of a licensed biological product as a manufacturer, packer, distributor, shared manufacturer, joint manufacturer, or any other participant involved in divided manufacturing. To avoid unnecessary duplication in the submission to FDA of reports required by paragraphs (c)(1)(i) and (c)(1)(ii) of this section, obligations of persons other than the applicant of the final biological product may be met by submission of all reports of serious adverse experiences to the applicant of the final product. If a person elects to submit adverse experience reports to the applicant rather than to FDA, the person must submit, by any appropriate means, each report to the applicant within 5 calendar days of initial receipt of the information by the person, and the applicant must then comply with the requirements of this section. Under this circumstance, a person who elects to submit reports to the applicant of the final product shall maintain a record of this action which must include:

(A) A copy of all adverse biological product experience reports submitted to the applicant of the final product;

(B) The date the report was received by the person;

(C) The date the report was submitted to the applicant of the final product; and—

(D) The name and address of the applicant of the final product.

(2) *Periodic adverse experience reports.* (i) The applicant must report each adverse experience not reported under paragraph (c)(1)(i) of this section at quarterly intervals, for 3 years from the date of issuance of the biologics license, and then at annual intervals. The applicant must submit each quarterly report within 30 days of the close of the quarter (the first quarter beginning on the date of issuance of the biologics license) and each annual report within 60 days of the anniversary date of the issuance of the biologics license. Upon written notice, FDA may extend or reestablish the requirement that an applicant submit quarterly reports, or require that the applicant submit reports under this section at different times than those stated. Followup information to adverse experiences submitted in a periodic report may be submitted in the next periodic report.

(ii) Each periodic report is required to contain:

(A) *Descriptive information. (1)* A narrative summary and analysis of the information in the report;

(2) An analysis of the 15-day Alert reports submitted during the reporting interval (all 15-day Alert reports being appropriately referenced by the applicant's patient identifi-

cation code for nonvaccine biological product reports or by the unique case identification number for vaccine reports, adverse reaction term(s), and date of submission to FDA);

(3) A history of actions taken since the last report because of adverse experiences (for example, labeling changes or studies initiated);

(4) An index consisting of a line listing of the applicant's patient identification code for nonvaccine biological product reports or by the unique case identification number for vaccine reports and adverse reaction term(s) for ICSRs submitted under paragraph (c)(2)(ii)(B) of this section; and

(B) *ICSRs for serious, expected and, nonserious adverse experiences.* An ICSR for each adverse experience not reported under paragraph (c)(1)(i) of this section (all serious, expected and nonserious adverse experiences). All such ICSRs must be submitted to FDA (either individually or in one or more batches) within the timeframe specified in paragraph (c)(2)(i) of this section. ICSRs must only be submitted to FDA once.

(iii) Periodic reporting, except for information regarding 15-day Alert reports, does not apply to adverse experience information obtained from postmarketing studies (whether or not conducted under an investigational new drug application), from reports in the scientific literature, and from foreign marketing experience.

(d) *Scientific literature.* A 15-day Alert report based on information in the scientific literature must be accompanied by a copy of the published article. The 15-day Alert reporting requirements in paragraph (c)(1)(i) of this section (i.e., serious, unexpected adverse experiences) apply only to reports found in scientific and medical journals either as case reports or as the result of a formal clinical trial.

(e) *Postmarketing studies.* Applicants are not required to submit a 15-day Alert report under paragraph (c) of this section for an adverse experience obtained from a postmarketing clinical study (whether or not conducted under a biological investigational new drug application) unless the applicant concludes that there is a reasonable possibility that the product caused the adverse experience.

(f) *Information reported on ICSRs for nonvaccine biological products.* ICSRs for nonvaccine biological products include the following information:

(1) *Patient information.*

(i) Patient identification code;

(ii) Patient age at the time of adverse experience, or date of birth;

(iii) Patient gender; and

(iv) Patient weight.

(2) *Adverse experience.*

(i) Outcome attributed to adverse experience;

(ii) Date of adverse experience;

(iii) Date of report;

(iv) Description of adverse experience (including a concise medical narrative);

(v) Adverse experience term(s);

(vi) Description of relevant tests, including dates and laboratory data; and

(vii) Other relevant patient history, including preexisting medical conditions.

(3) *Suspect medical product(s).*

(i) Name;

(ii) Dose, frequency, and route of administration used;

(iii) Therapy dates;

(iv) Diagnosis for use (indication);

(v) Whether the product is a combination product as defined in §3.2(e) of this chapter;

(vi) Whether the product is a prescription or nonprescription product;

(vii) Whether adverse experience abated after product use stopped or dose reduced;

(viii) Whether adverse experience reappeared after eintroduction of the product;

(ix) Lot number;

(x) Expiration date;

(xi) National Drug Code (NDC) number, or other unique identifier; and

(xii) Concomitant medical products and therapy dates.

(4) *Initial reporter information.*

(i) Name, address, and telephone number;

(ii) Whether the initial reporter is a health care professional; and

(iii) Occupation, if a health care professional.

(5) *Applicant information.*

(i) Applicant name and contact office address;

(ii) Telephone number;

(iii) Report source, such as spontaneous, literature, or study;

(iv) Date the report was received by applicant;

(v) Application number and type;

(vi) Whether the ICSR is a 15-day "Alert report";

(vii) Whether the ICSR is an initial report or followup report; and

(viii) Unique case identification number, which must be the same in the initial report and any subsequent followup report(s).

(g) *Information reported on ICSRs for vaccine products.* ICSRs for vaccine products include the following information:

(1) *Patient information.*

(i) Patient name, address, telephone number;

(ii) Patient age at the time of vaccination, or date of birth;

(iii) Patient gender; and

(iv) Patient birth weight for children under age 5.

(2) *Adverse experience.*

(i) Outcome attributed to adverse experience;

(ii) Date and time of adverse experience;

(iii) Date of report;

(iv) Description of adverse experience (including a concise medical narrative);

(v) Adverse experience term(s);

(vi) Illness at the time of vaccination;

(vii) Description of relevant tests, including dates and laboratory data; and

(viii) Other relevant patient history, including preexisting medical conditions.

(3) *Suspect medical product(s), including vaccines administered on the same date.*

(i) Name;

(ii) Dose, frequency, and route or site of administration used;

(iii) Number of previous vaccine doses;

(iv) Vaccination date(s) and time(s);

(v) Diagnosis for use (indication);

(vi) Whether the product is a combination product (as defined in §3.2(e) of this chapter);

(vii) Whether the adverse experience abated after product use stopped or dose reduced;

(viii) Whether the adverse experience reappeared after reintroduction of the product;

(ix) Lot number;

(x) Expiration date;

(xi) National Drug Code (NDC) number, or other unique identifier; and

(xii) Concomitant medical products and therapy dates.

(4) *Vaccine(s) administered in the 4 weeks prior to the vaccination date.*

(i) Name of vaccine;

(ii) Manufacturer;

(iii) Lot number;

(iv) Route or site of administration;

(v) Date given; and

(vi) Number of previous doses.

(5) *Initial reporter information.*

(i) Name, address, and telephone number;

(ii) Whether the initial reporter is a health care professional; and

(iii) Occupation, if a health care professional.

(6) *Facility and personnel where vaccine was administered.*

(i) Name of person who administered vaccine;

(ii) Name of responsible physician at facility where vaccine was administered; and

(iii) Name, address (including city, county, and state), and telephone number of facility where vaccine was administered.

(7) *Applicant information.*

(i) Applicant name and contact office address;

(ii) Telephone number;

(iii) Report source, such as spontaneous, literature, or study;

(iv) Date received by applicant;

(v) Application number and type;

(vi) Whether the ICSR is a 15-day "Alert report";

(vii) Whether the ICSR is an initial report or followup report; and

(viii) Unique case identification number, which must be the same in the initial report and any subsequent followup report(s).

(h) *Electronic format for submissions.* (1) Safety report submissions, including ICSRs, ICSR attachments, and the descriptive information in periodic reports, must be in an electronic format that FDA can process, review, and archive. FDA will issue guidance on how to provide the electronic submission (e.g., method of transmission, media, file formats, preparation and organization of files).

(2) Persons subject to the requirements of paragraph (c) of this section may request, in writing, a temporary waiver of the requirements in paragraph (h)(1) of this section. These waivers will be granted on a limited basis for good cause shown. FDA will issue guidance on requesting a waiver of the requirements in paragraph (h)(1) of this section. Requests for waivers must be submitted in accordance with §600.90.

(i) *Multiple reports.* An applicant should not include in reports under this section any adverse experience that occurred in clinical trials if they were previously submitted as part of the biologics license application. If a report refers to more than one biological product marketed by an applicant, the applicant should submit the report to the biologics license application for the product listed first in the report.

(j) *Patient privacy.* For nonvaccine biological products, an applicant should not include in reports under this section the names and addresses of individual patients; instead, the applicant should assign a unique code for identification of the patient. The applicant should include the name of the reporter from whom the information was received as part of the initial reporter information, even when the reporter is the patient. The names of patients, health care professionals, hospitals, and geographical identifiers in adverse experience reports are not releasable to the public under FDA's public information regulations in part 20 of this chapter. For vaccine adverse experience reports, these data will become part of the CDC Privacy Act System 09-20-0136, "Epidemiologic Studies and Surveillance of Disease Problems." Information identifying the person who received the vaccine or that person's legal representative will not be made available to the public, but may be available to the vaccinee or legal representative.

(k) *Recordkeeping.* The applicant must maintain for a period of 10 years records of all adverse experiences known to the applicant, including raw data and any correspondence relating to the adverse experiences.

(l) *Revocation of biologics license.* If an applicant fails to establish and maintain records and make reports required under this section with respect to a licensed biological product, FDA may revoke the biologics license for such a product in accordance with the procedures of §601.5 of this chapter.

(m) *Exemptions.* Manufacturers of the following listed products are not required to submit adverse experience reports under this section:

(1) Whole blood or components of whole blood.

(2) In vitro diagnostic products, including assay systems for the detection of antibodies or antigens to retroviruses. These products are subject to the reporting requirements for devices.

(n) *Disclaimer.* A report or information submitted by an applicant under this section (and any release by FDA of that report or information) does not necessarily reflect a conclusion by the applicant or FDA that the report or information constitutes an admission that the biological product caused or contributed to an adverse effect. An applicant need not admit, and may deny, that the report or information submitted under this section constitutes an admission that the biological product caused or contributed to an adverse effect. For purposes of this provision, this paragraph also includes any person reporting under paragraph (c)(1)(iii) of this section.

[59 FR 54042, Oct. 27, 1994, as amended at 62 FR 34168, June 25, 1997; 62 FR 52252, Oct. 7, 1997; 63 FR 14612, Mar. 26, 1998; 64 FR 56449, Oct. 20, 1999; 70 FR 14982, Mar. 24, 2005; 79 FR 33090, June 10, 2014]

§600.81   Distribution reports.

(a) *Reporting requirements.* The applicant must submit to the Center for Biologics Evaluation and Research or the Center for Drug Evaluation and Research, information about the quantity of the product distributed under the biologics license, including the quantity distributed to distributors. The interval between distribution reports must be 6 months. Upon written notice, FDA may require that the applicant submit distribution reports under this section at times other than every 6 months. The distribution report must consist of the bulk lot number (from which the final container was filled), the fill lot numbers for the total number of dosage units of each strength or potency distributed (c.g., fifty thousand per 10-milliliter vials), the label lot number (if different from fill lot number), labeled date of expiration, number of doses in fill lot/label lot, date of release of fill lot/label lot for distribution at that time. If any significant amount of a fill lot/label lot is returned, include this information. Disclosure of financial or pricing data is not required. As needed, FDA may require submission of more detailed product distribution information. Upon written notice, FDA may require that the applicant submit reports under this section at times other than those stated. Requests by an applicant to submit reports at times other than those stated should be made as a request for a waiver under §600.90

(b)(1) *Electronic format.* Except as provided for in paragraph (b)(2) of this section, the distribution reports required under paragraph (a) of this section must be submitted to the Agency in an electronic format that FDA can process, review, and archive. FDA will issue guidance on how to provide the electronic submission (e.g., method of transmission, media, file formats, preparation and organization of files).

(2) *Waivers.* An applicant may request, in writing, a temporary waiver of the requirements in paragraph (b)(1) of this section. These waivers will be granted on a limited basis for good cause shown. FDA will issue guidance on requesting a waiver of the requirements in paragraph (b)(1) of this section. Requests for waivers must be submitted in accordance with §600.90.

[59 FR 54042, Oct. 27, 1994, as amended at 64 FR 56449, Oct. 20, 1999; 70 FR 14983, Mar. 24, 2005; 79 FR 33091, June 10, 2014]

§600.82 Notification of a permanent discontinuance or an interruption in manufacturing.

(a) *Notification of a permanent discontinuance or an interruption in manufacturing.* (1) An applicant of a biological product, other than blood or blood components for transfusion, which is licensed under section 351 of the Public Health Service Act, and which may be dispensed only under prescription under section 503(b)(1) of the Federal Food, Drug, and Cosmetic Act (21 U.S.C. 353(b)(1)), must notify FDA in writing of a permanent discontinuance of manufacture of the biological product or an interruption in manufacturing of the biological product that is likely to lead to a meaningful disruption in supply of that biological product in the United States if:

(i) The biological product is life supporting, life sustaining, or intended for use in the prevention or treatment of a debilitating disease or condition, including any such biological product used in emergency medical care or during surgery; and

(ii) The biological product is not a radiopharmaceutical biological product.

(2) An applicant of blood or blood components for transfusion, which is licensed under section 351 of the Public Health Service Act, and which may be dispensed only

under prescription under section 503(b) of the Federal Food, Drug, and Cosmetic Act, must notify FDA in writing of a permanent discontinuance of manufacture of any product listed in its license or an interruption in manufacturing of any such product that is likely to lead to a significant disruption in supply of that product in the United States if:

(i) The product is life supporting, life sustaining, or intended for use in the prevention or treatment of a debilitating disease or condition, including any such product used in emergency medical care or during surgery; and

(ii) The applicant is a manufacturer of a significant percentage of the U.S. blood supply.

(b) *Submission and timing of notification.* Notifications required by paragraph (a) of this section must be submitted to FDA electronically in a format that FDA can process, review, and archive:

(1) At least 6 months prior to the date of the permanent discontinuance or interruption in manufacturing; or

(2) If 6 months' advance notice is not possible because the permanent discontinuance or interruption in manufacturing was not reasonably anticipated 6 months in advance, as soon as practicable thereafter, but in no case later than 5 business days after such a permanent discontinuance or interruption in manufacturing occurs.

(c) *Information included in notification.* Notifications required by paragraph (a) of this section must include the following information:

(1) The name of the biological product subject to the notification, including the National Drug Code for such biological product, or an alternative standard for identification and labeling that has been recognized as acceptable by the Center Director;

(2) The name of the applicant of the biological product;

(3) Whether the notification relates to a permanent discontinuance of the biological product or an interruption in manufacturing of the biological product;

(4) A description of the reason for the permanent discontinuance or interruption in manufacturing; and

(5) The estimated duration of the interruption in manufacturing.

(d)(1) *Public list of biological product shortages.* FDA will maintain a publicly available list of biological products that are determined by FDA to be in shortage. This biological product shortages list will include the following information:

(i) The names and National Drug Codes for such biological products, or the alternative standards for identification and labeling that have been recognized as acceptable by the Center Director;

(ii) The name of each applicant for such biological products;

(iii) The reason for the shortage, as determined by FDA, selecting from the following categories: Requirements related to complying with good manufacturing practices; regulatory delay; shortage of an active ingredient; shortage of an inactive ingredient component; discontinuation of the manufacture of the biological product; delay in shipping of the biological product; demand increase for the biological product; or other reason; and

(iv) The estimated duration of the shortage.

(2) *Confidentiality.* FDA may choose not to make information collected to implement this paragraph available on the biological product shortages list or available under section 506C(c) of the Federal Food, Drug, and Cosmetic Act (21 U.S.C. 356c(c)) if FDA determines that disclosure of such information would adversely affect the public health (such as by increasing the possibility of hoarding or other disruption of the availability of the biological product to patients). FDA will also not provide information on the public shortages list or under section 506C(c) of the Federal Food, Drug, and Cosmetic Act that is protected by 18 U.S.C. 1905 or 5 U.S.C. 552(b)(4), including trade secrets and commercial or financial information that is considered confidential or privileged under §20.61 of this chapter.

(e) Noncompliance letters. If an applicant fails to submit a notification as required under paragraph (a) of this section and in accordance with paragraph (b) of this section,

FDA will issue a letter to the applicant informing it of such failure.

(1) Not later than 30 calendar days after the issuance of such a letter, the applicant must submit to FDA a written response setting forth the basis for noncompliance and providing the required notification under paragraph (a) of this section and including the information required under paragraph (c) of this section; and

(2) Not later than 45 calendar days after the issuance of a letter under this paragraph, FDA will make the letter and the applicant's response to the letter public, unless, after review of the applicant's response, FDA determines that the applicant had a reasonable basis for not notifying FDA as required under paragraph (a) of this section.

(f) *Definitions.* The following definitions of terms apply to this section:

Biological product shortage or shortage means a period of time when the demand or projected demand for the biological product within the United States exceeds the supply of the biological product.

Intended for use in the prevention or treatment of a debilitating disease or condition means a biological product intended for use in the prevention or treatment of a disease or condition associated with mortality or morbidity that has a substantial impact on day-to-day functioning.

Life supporting or life sustaining means a biological product that is essential to, or that yields information that is essential to, the restoration or continuation of a bodily function important to the continuation of human life.

Meaningful disruption means a change in production that is reasonably likely to lead to a reduction in the supply of a biological product by a manufacturer that is more than negligible and affects the ability of the manufacturer to fill orders or meet expected demand for its product, and does not include interruptions in manufacturing due to matters such as routine maintenance or insignificant changes in manufacturing so long as the manufacturer expects to resume operations in a short period of time.

Significant disruption means a change in production that

is reasonably likely to lead to a reduction in the supply of blood or blood components by a manufacturer that substantially affects the ability of the manufacturer to fill orders or meet expected demand for its product, and does not include interruptions in manufacturing due to matters such as routine maintenance or insignificant changes in manufacturing so long as the manufacturer expects to resume operations in a short period of time.

[80 FR 38939, July 8, 2015]

§600.90   Waivers.

(a) An applicant may ask the Food and Drug Administration to waive under this section any requirement that applies to the applicant under §§600.80 and 600.81. A waiver request under this section is required to be submitted with supporting documentation. The waiver request is required to contain one of the following:

(1) An explanation why the applicant's compliance with the requirement is unnecessary or cannot be achieved,

(2) A description of an alternative submission that satisfies the purpose of the requirement, or

(3) Other information justifying a waiver.

(b) FDA may grant a waiver if it finds one of the following:

(1) The applicant's compliance with the requirement is unnecessary or cannot be achieved,

(2) The applicant's alternative submission satisfies the requirement, or

(3) The applicant's submission otherwise justifies a waiver.

[59 FR 54042, Oct. 27, 1994, as amended at 79 FR 33092, June 10, 2014]

Notes:

Notes

Part 601

The Code of Federal Regulations
Title 21 – Food and Drugs

Part 601
LICENSING

Printed by GMP Publications, Inc.
Tel: 866-544-9007 or 856-810-7331
Fax: 866-544-9002
http://www.gmppublications.com
sales@gmppublications.com

PART 601--LICENSING

Subpart A--General Provisions

Subpart B [Reserved]

Subpart C--Biologics Licensing

Subpart D--Diagnostic Radiopharmaceuticals

Subpart E--Accelerated Approval of Biological Products for Serious or Life-Threatening Illnesses

Subpart F--Confidentiality of Information

Subpart G--Postmarketing Studies

Subpart H--Approval of Biological Products When Human Efficacy Studies Are Not Ethical or Feasible

Authority: 15 U.S.C. 1451-1561; 21 U.S.C. 321, 351, 352, 353, 355, 356b, 360, 360c-360f, 360h-360j, 371, 374, 379e, 381; 42 U.S.C. 216, 241, 262, 263, 264; sec 122, Pub. L. 105-115, 111 Stat. 2322 (21 U.S.C. 355 note).

Source: 38 FR 32052, Nov. 20, 1973, unless otherwise noted.

Cross References: For U.S. Customs Service regulations relating to viruses, serums, and toxins, see 19 CFR 12.21-12.23. For U.S. Postal Service regulations relating to the admissibility to the United States mails see parts 124 and 125 of the Domestic Mail Manual, that is incorporated by reference in 39 CFR part 111.

Subpart A--General Provisions

§601.2 Applications for biologics licenses; procedures for filing.

(a) *General.* To obtain a biologics license under section 351 of the Public Health Service Act for any biological product, the manufacturer shall submit an application to the Director, Center for Biologics Evaluation and Research or the Director, Center for Drug Evaluation and Research (see mailing addresses in §600.2(a) or (b) of this chapter), on forms prescribed for such purposes, and shall submit data derived from nonclinical laboratory and clinical studies which demonstrate that the manufactured product meets prescribed requirements of safety, purity, and potency; with respect to each nonclinical laboratory study, either a statement that the study was conducted in compliance with the requirements set forth in part 58 of this chapter, or, if the study was not conducted in compliance with such regulations, a brief statement of the reason for the noncompliance; statements regarding each clinical investigation involving human subjects contained in the application, that it either was conducted in compliance with tho roquiromonts for institutional review set forth in part 56 of this chapter; or was not subject to such requirements in accordance with §56.104 or §56.105, and was conducted in compliance with requirements for informed consent set forth in part 50 of this chapter. A full description of manufacturing methods; data establishing stability of the product through the dating period; sample(s) representative of the product for introduction or delivery for introduction into interstate commerce; summaries of results of tests performed on the lot(s) represented by the submitted sample(s); specimens of the labels, enclosures, and containers, and if applicable, any Medication Guide required under part 208 of this chapter proposed to be used for the product; and the address of each location involved in the manufacture of the biological product shall be listed in the biologics license application. The applicant shall also include a financial certification or disclosure statement(s) or both for clinical investigators as required by part 54 of this chapter. An application for a biologics license shall not be considered as filed until all pertinent information and data have been received by the Food and Drug Administration. The applicant shall also include either a claim for categorical exclusion under §25.30 or §25.31 of this chapter or an environmental assessment under §25.40 of this chapter. The applicant, or the applicant's attorney, agent, or other authorized official shall sign the application. An application for any of the following specified categories of biological products subject to licensure shall be handled as set forth in paragraph (c) of this section:

(1) Therapeutic DNA plasmid products;

(2) Therapeutic synthetic peptide products of 40 or fewer amino acids;

(3) Monoclonal antibody products for in vivo use; and

(4) Therapeutic recombinant DNA-derived products.

(b) [Reserved]

(c)(1) To obtain marketing approval for a biological product subject to licensure which is a therapeutic DNA plasmid product, therapeutic synthetic peptide product of 40 or fewer amino acids, monoclonal antibody product for in vivo use, or therapeutic recombinant DNA-derived product, an applicant shall submit a biologics license application in accordance with paragraph (a) of this section except that the following sections in parts 600 through 680 of this chapter shall not be applicable to such products: §§600.10(b) and (c), 600.11, 600.12, 600.13, 610.53, and 610.62 of this chapter.

(2) To the extent that the requirements in this paragraph (c) conflict with other requirements in this subchapter (except for those products described in paragraph (b) of this section for which a new drug application is required), this paragraph (c) shall supersede other requirements.

(d) Approval of a biologics license application or issuance of a biologics license shall constitute a determination that the establishment(s) and the product meet applicable requirements to ensure the continued safety, purity, and potency of such products. Applicable requirements for the maintenance of establishments for the manufacture of a product subject to this section shall include but not be limited to the good manufacturing practice requirements set forth in parts 210, 211, 600, 606, and 820 of this chapter.

(e) Any establishment and product license for a biological product issued under section 351 of the Public Health Service Act (42 U.S.C. 201 et seq.) that has not been revoked or suspended as of December 20, 1999, shall constitute an approved biologics license application in effect under the same terms and conditions set forth in such product license and such portions of the establishment license relating to such product.

(f) *Withdrawal from sale of approved biological products.* A holder of a biologics license application (BLA) must report to FDA, in accordance with the requirements of Sec. Sec. 207.61 and 207.65, the withdrawal from sale of an approved biological product. The information must be submitted to FDA within 30 working days of the biological product's withdrawal from sale. The following information must be submitted: The holder's name; product name; BLA number; the National Drug Code; and the date on which the product is expected to be no longer in commercial distribution. The reason for the withdrawal of the biological product is requested but not required to be submitted.

[64 FR 56450, Oct. 20, 1999, as amended at 70 FR 14983, Mar. 24, 2005; 80 FR 18092, Apr. 3, 2015; 80 FR 37974, July 2, 2015; 81 FR 60221, Aug. 31, 2016]

§601.3   Complete response letter to the applicant.

(a) Complete response letter. The Food and Drug Administration will send the biologics license applicant or supplement applicant a complete response letter if the agency determines that it will not approve the biologics license application or supplement in its present form.

(1) Description of specific deficiencies. A complete response letter will describe all of the deficiencies that the

agency has identified in a biologics license application or supplement, except as stated in paragraph (a)(2) of this section.

(2) Inadequate data. If FDA determines, after a biologics license application or supplement is filed, that the data submitted are inadequate to support approval, the agency might issue a complete response letter without first conducting required inspections, testing submitted product lots, and/or reviewing proposed product labeling.

(3) Recommendation of actions for approval. When possible, a complete response letter will recommend actions that the applicant might take to place its biologics license application or supplement in condition for approval.

(b) Applicant actions. After receiving a complete response letter, the biologics license applicant or supplement applicant must take either of the following actions:

(1) Resubmission. Resubmit the application or supplement, addressing all deficiencies identified in the complete response letter.

(2) Withdrawal. Withdraw the application or supplement. A decision to withdraw the application or supplement is without prejudice to a subsequent submission.

(c) Failure to take action. (1) FDA may consider a biologics license applicant or supplement applicant's failure to either resubmit or withdraw the application or supplement within 1 year after issuance of a complete response letter to be a request by the applicant to withdraw the application or supplement, unless the applicant has requested an extension of time in which to resubmit the application or supplement. FDA will grant any reasonable request for such an extension. FDA may consider an applicant's failure to resubmit the application or supplement within the extended time period or request an additional extension to be a request by the applicant to withdraw the application.

(2) If FDA considers an applicant's failure to take action in accordance with paragraph (c)(1) of this section to be a request to withdraw the application, the agency will notify the applicant in writing. The applicant will have 30 days from the date of the notification to explain why the applica-

tion or supplement should not be withdrawn and to request an extension of time in which to resubmit the application or supplement. FDA will grant any reasonable request for an extension. If the applicant does not respond to the notification within 30 days, the application or supplement will be deemed to be withdrawn.

[73 FR 39611, July 10, 2008]

§601.4   Issuance and denial of license.

(a) A biologics license shall be issued upon a determination by the Director, Center for Biologics Evaluation and Research that the establishment(s) and the product meet the applicable requirements established in this chapter. A biologics license shall be valid until suspended or revoked.

(b) If the Commissioner determines that the establishment or product does not meet the requirements established in this chapter, the biologics license application shall be denied and the applicant shall be informed of the grounds for, and of an opportunity for a hearing on, the decision. If the applicant so requests, the Commissioner shall issue a notice of opportunity for hearing on the matter pursuant to §12.21(b) of this chapter.

[42 FR 4718, Jan. 25, 1977, as amended at 42 FR 15676, Mar. 22, 1977; 42 FR 19142, Apr. 12, 1977; 64 FR 56450, Oct. 20, 1999; 70 FR 14983, Mar. 24, 2005]

§601.5   Revocation of license.

(a) A biologics license shall be revoked upon application of the manufacturer giving notice of intention to discontinue the manufacture of all products manufactured under such license or to discontinue the manufacture of a particular product for which a license is held and waiving an opportunity for a hearing on the matter.

(b)(1) The Commissioner shall notify the licensed manufacturer of the intention to revoke the biologics license, setting forth the grounds for, and offering an opportunity for a hearing on the proposed revocation if the Commissioner finds any of the following:

(i) Authorized Food and Drug Administration employees after reasonable efforts have been unable to gain access to an establishment or a location for the purpose of carrying out the inspection required under §600.21 of this chapter,

(ii) Manufacturing of products or of a product has been discontinued to an extent that a meaningful inspection or evaluation cannot be made,

(iii) The manufacturer has failed to report a change as required by §601.12 of this chapter,

(iv) The establishment or any location thereof, or the product for which the license has been issued, fails to conform to the applicable standards established in the license and in this chapter designed to ensure the continued safety, purity, and potency of the manufactured product,

(v) The establishment or the manufacturing methods have been so changed as to require a new showing that the establishment or product meets the requirements established in this chapter in order to protect the public health, or

(vi) The licensed product is not safe and effective for all of its intended uses or is misbranded with respect to any such use.

(2) Except as provided in §601.6 of this chapter, or in cases involving willfulness, the notification required in this paragraph shall provide a reasonable period for the licensed manufacturer to demonstrate or achieve compliance with the requirements of this chapter, before proceedings will be instituted for the revocation of the license. If compliance is not demonstrated or achieved and the licensed manufacturer does not waive the opportunity for a hearing, the Commissioner shall issue a notice of opportunity for hearing on the matter under §12.21(b) of this chapter.

[64 FR 56451, Oct. 20, 1999]

§601.6   Suspension of license.

(a) Whenever the Commissioner has reasonable grounds to believe that any of the grounds for revocation of a license exist and that by reason thereof there is a danger to health, the Commissioner may notify the licensed manufacturer that the biologics license is suspended and require that the licensed manufacturer do the following:

(1) Notify the selling agents and distributors to whom such product or products have been delivered of such suspension, and

(2) Furnish to the Director, Center for Biologics Evaluation and Research, complete records of such deliveries and notice of suspension.

(b) Upon suspension of a license, the Commissioner shall either:

(1) Proceed under the provisions of §601.5(b) of this chapter to revoke the license, or

(2) If the licensed manufacturer agrees, hold revocation in abeyance pending resolution of the matters involved.

[64 FR 56451, Oct. 20, 1999, as amended at 70 FR 14983, Mar. 24, 2005]

§601.7   Procedure for hearings.

(a) A notice of opportunity for hearing, notice of appearance and request for hearing, and grant or denial of hearing for a biological drug pursuant to this part, for which the exemption from the Federal Food, Drug, and Cosmetic Act in §310.4 of this chapter has been revoked, shall be subject to the provisions of §314.200 of this chapter except to the extent that the notice of opportunity for hearing on the matter issued pursuant to §12.21(b) of this chapter specifically provides otherwise.

(b) Hearings pursuant to §§601.4 through 601.6 shall be governed by part 12 of this chapter.

(c) When a license has been suspended pursuant to §601.6 and a hearing request has been granted, the hearing shall proceed on an expedited basis.

[42 FR 4718, Jan. 25, 1977, as amended at 42 FR 15676, Mar. 22, 1977; 42 FR 19143, Apr. 12, 1977]

§601.8   Publication of revocation.

The Commissioner, following revocation of a biologics license under 21 CFR 601.5(b), will publish a notice in the Federal Register with a statement of the specific grounds for the revocation.

[74 FR 20585, May 5, 2009]

§601.9   Licenses; reissuance.

(a) *Compliance with requirements.* A biologics license, previously suspended or revoked, may be reissued orreinstated upon a showing of compliance with requirements and upon such inspection and examination as may be considered necessary by the Director, Center for Biologics Evaluation and Research or the Director, Center for Drug Evaluation and Research.

(b) *Exclusion of noncomplying location.* A biologics license, excluding a location or locations that fail to comply with the requirements in this chapter, may be issued without further application and concurrently with the suspension or revocation of the license for noncompliance at the excluded location or locations.

(c) *Exclusion of noncomplying product(s).* In the case of multiple products included under a single biologics license application, a biologics license may be issued, excluding the noncompliant product(s), without further application and concurrently with the suspension or revocation of the biologics license for a noncompliant product(s).

[64 FR 56451, Oct. 20, 1999, as amended at 70 FR 14983, Mar. 24, 2005]

Subpart B [Reserved]

Subpart C--Biologics Licensing

§601.12   Changes to an approved application.

(a) *General.* (1) As provided by this section, an applicant must inform the Food and Drug Administration (FDA) about each change in the product, production process, quality controls, equipment, facilities, responsible personnel, or labeling established in the approved license application(s).

(2) Before distributing a product made using a change, an applicant must assess the effects of the change and demonstrate through appropriate validation and/or other clinical and/or nonclinical laboratory studies the lack of adverse effect of the change on the identity, strength, quality, purity, or potency of the product as they may relate to the safety or effectiveness of the product.

(3) Notwithstanding the requirements of paragraphs (b), (c), and (f) of this section, an applicant must make a change provided for in those paragraphs in accordance with a regulation or guidance that provides for a less burdensome notification of the change (for example, by submission of a supplement that does not require approval prior to distribution of the product or in an annual report).

(4) The applicant must promptly revise all promotional labeling and advertising to make it consistent with any labeling change implemented in accordance with paragraphs (f)(1) and (f)(2) of this section.

(5) A supplement or annual report must include a list of all changes contained in the supplement or annual report. For supplements, this list must be provided in the cover letter.

(b) *Changes requiring supplement submission and approval prior to distribution of the product made using the change (major changes).* (1) A supplement shall besubmitted for any change in the product, production process, quality controls, equipment, facilities, or responsible personnel that has a substantial potential to have an adverse effect on the identity, strength, quality, purity, or potency of the product as they may relate to the safety or effectiveness of the product.

(2) These changes include, but are not limited to:

(i) Except as provided in paragraphs (c) and (d) of this section, changes in the qualitative or quantitative formulation, including inactive ingredients, or in the specifications provided in the approved application;

(ii) Changes requiring completion of an appropriate

human study to demonstrate the equivalence of the identity, strength, quality, purity, or potency of the product as they may relate to the safety or effectiveness of the product;

(iii) Changes in the virus or adventitious agent removal or inactivation method(s);

(iv) Changes in the source material or cell line;

(v) Establishment of a new master cell bank or seed; and

(vi) Changes which may affect product sterility assurance, such as changes in product or component sterilization method(s), or an addition, deletion, or substitution of steps in an aseptic processing operation.

(3) The applicant must obtain approval of the supplement from FDA prior to distribution of the product made using the change. Except for submissions under paragraph (e) of this section, the following shall be contained in the supplement:

(i) A detailed description of the proposed change;

(ii) The product(s) involved;

(iii) The manufacturing site(s) or area(s) affected;

(iv) A description of the methods used and studies performed to evaluate the effect of the change on the identity, strength, quality, purity, or potency of the product as they may relate to the safety or effectiveness of the product;

(v) The data derived from such studies;

(vi) Relevant validation protocols and data; and

(vii) A reference list of relevant standard operating procedures (SOP's).

(4) An applicant may ask FDA to expedite its review of a supplement for public health reasons or if a delay in making the change described in it would impose an extraordinary hardship on the applicant. Such a supplement and its mailing cover should be plainly marked: "Prior Approval Supplement-Expedited Review Requested".

(c) *Changes requiring supplement submission at least 30 days prior to distribution of the product made using the change.* (1) A supplement shall be submitted for any change in the product, production process, quality controls, equipment, facilities, or responsible personnel that has a moderate potential to have an adverse effect on the identity, strength, quality, purity, or potency of the product as they may relate to the safety or effectiveness of the product. The supplement shall be labeled "Supplement--Changes Being Effected in 30 Days" or, if applicable under paragraph (c)(5) of this section, "Supplement--Changes Being Effected."

(2) These changes include, but are not limited to:

(i) [Reserved]

(ii) An increase or decrease in production scale during finishing steps that involves different equipment; and

(iii) Replacement of equipment with that of similar, but not identical, design and operating principle that does not affect the process methodology or process operating parameters.

(iv) Relaxation of an acceptance criterion or deletion of a test to comply with an official compendium that is consistent with FDA statutory and regulatory requirements.

(3) Pending approval of the supplement by FDA, and except as provided in paragraph (c)(5) of this section, distribution of the product made using the change may begin not less than 30 days after receipt of the supplement by FDA. The information listed in paragraph (b)(3)(i) through (b)(3)(vii) of this section shall be contained in the supplement.

(4) If within 30 days following FDA's receipt of the supplement, FDA informs the applicant that either:

(i) The change requires approval prior to distribution of the product in accordance with paragraph (b) of this section; or

(ii) Any of the information required under paragraph (c)(3) of this section is missing; the applicant shall not distribute the product made using the change until FDA determines that compliance with this section is achieved.

(5) In certain circumstances, FDA may determine that, based on experience with a particular type of change, the supplement for such change is usually complete and provides the proper information, and on particular assurances that the proposed change has been appropriately submitted, the product made using the change may be

distributed immediately upon receipt of the supplement by FDA. These circumstances may include substantial similarity with a type of change regularly involving a "Supplement--Changes Being Effected" supplement or a situation in which the applicant presents evidence that the proposed change has been validated in accordance with an approved protocol for such change under paragraph (e) of this section.

(6) If the agency disapproves the supplemental application, it may order the manufacturer to cease distribution of the products made with the manufacturing change.

(d) *Changes to be described in an annual report (minor changes).* (1) Changes in the product, production process, quality controls, equipment, facilities, or responsible personnel that have a minimal potential to have an adverse effect on the identity, strength, quality, purity, or potency of the product as they may relate to the safety or effectiveness of the product shall be documented by the applicant in an annual report submitted each year within 60 days of the anniversary date of approval of the application. The Director, Center for Biologics Evaluation and Research, may approve a written request for an alternative date to combine annual reports for multiple approved applications into a single annual report submission.

(2) These changes include, but are not limited to:

(i) Any change made to comply with a change to an official compendium, except a change described in paragraph (c)(2)(iv) of this section, that is consistent with FDA statutory and regulatory requirements.

(ii) The deletion or reduction of an ingredient intended only to affect the color of the product, except that a change intended only to affect Blood Grouping Reagents requires supplement submission and approval prior to distribution of the product made using the change in accordance with the requirements set forth in paragraph (b) of this section;

(iii) An extension of an expiration dating period based upon full shelf life data on production batches obtained from a protocol approved in the application;

(iv) A change within the container closure system for a nonsterile product, based upon a showing of equivalency to the approved system under a protocol approved in the application or published in an official compendium;

(v) A change in the size and/or shape of a container containing the same number of dosage units for a nonsterile solid dosage form product, without a change from one container closure system to another;

(vi) The addition by embossing, debossing, or engraving of a code imprint to a solid dosage form biological product other than a modified release dosage form, or a minor change in an existing code imprint; and

(vii) The addition or revision of an alternative analytical procedure that provides the same or increased assurance of the identity, strength, quality, purity, or potency of the material being tested as the analytical procedure described in the approved application, or deletion of an alternative analytical procedure.

(3) The following information for each change shall be contained in the annual report:

(i) A list of all products involved; and

(ii) A full description of the manufacturing and controls changes including: the manufacturing site(s) or area(s) involved; the date the change was made; a cross-reference to relevant validation protocols and/or SOP's; and relevant data from studies and tests performed to evaluate the effect of the change on the identity, strength, quality, purity, or potency of the product as they may relate to the safety or effectiveness of the product.

(iii) A statement by the holder of the approved application or license that the effects of the change have been assessed.

(4) The applicant shall submit the report to the FDA office responsible for reviewing the application. The report shall include all the information required under this paragraph for each change made during the annual reporting interval which ends on the anniversary date in the order in which they were implemented.

(e) An applicant may submit one or more protocols describing the specific tests and validation studies and acceptable limits to be achieved to demonstrate the lack of adverse effect for specified types of manufacturing changes on the identity, strength, quality, purity, or potency of the product as they may relate to the safety or effectiveness of the product. Any such protocols, or change to a protocol, shall be submitted as a supplement requiring approval from FDA prior to distribution of the product which, if approved, may justify a reduced reporting category for the particular change because the use of the protocol for that type of change reduces the potential risk of an adverse effect.

(f) *Labeling changes.* (1) Labeling changes requiring supplement submission--FDA approval must be obtained before distribution of the product with the labeling change. Except as described in paragraphs (f)(2) and (f)(3) of this section, an applicant shall submit a supplement describing a proposed change in the package insert, package label, container label, or, if applicable, a Medication Guide required under part 208 of this chapter, and include the information necessary to support the proposed change. An applicant cannot use paragraph (f)(2) of this section to make any change to the information required in §201.57(a) of this chapter. An applicant may report the minor changes to the information specified in paragraph (f)(3)(i)(D) of this section in an annual report. The supplement shall clearly highlight the proposed change in the labeling. The applicant shall obtain approval from FDA prior to distribution of the product with the labeling change.

(2) *Labeling changes requiring supplement submission--product with a labeling change that may be distributed before FDA approval.* (i) An applicant shall submit, at the time such change is made, a supplement for any change in the package insert, package label, or container label to reflect newly acquired information, except for changes to the package insert required in §201.57(a) of this chapter (which must be made under paragraph (f)(1) of this section), to accomplish any of the following:

(A) To add or strengthen a contraindication, warning, precaution, or adverse reaction for which the evidence of a causal association satisfies the standard for inclusion in the labeling under §201.57(c) of this chapter;

(B) To add or strengthen a statement about abuse, dependence, psychological effect, or overdosage;

(C) To add or strengthen an instruction about dosage and administration that is intended to increase the safety of the use of the product; and

(D) To delete false, misleading, or unsupported indications for use or claims for effectiveness.

(E) Any labeling change normally requiring a supplement submission and approval prior to distribution of the product that FDA specifically requests be submitted under this provision.

(ii) Pending approval of the supplement by FDA, the applicant may distribute a product with a package insert, package label, or container label bearing such change at the time the supplement is submitted. The supplement shall clearly identify the change being made and include necessary supporting data. The supplement and its mailing cover shall be plainly marked: "Special Labeling Supplement--Changes Being Effected."

(3) *Labeling changes requiring submission in an annual report.* (i) An applicant shall submit any final printed package insert, package label, container label, or Medication Guide required under part 208 of this chapter incorporating the following changes in an annual report submitted to FDA each year as provided in paragraph (d)(1) of this section:

(A) Editorial or similar minor changes;

(B) A change in the information on how the product is supplied that does not involve a change in the dosage strength or dosage form;

(C) A change in the information specified in §208.20(b)(8)(iii) and (b)(8)(iv) of this chapter for a Medication Guide; and

(D) A change to the information required in §201.57(a) of this chapter as follows:

(*1*) Removal of a listed section(s) specified in §201.57 (a)(5) of this chapter; and

(*2*) Changes to the most recent revision date of the labeling as specified in § 201.57(a)(15) of this chapter.

(E) A change made pursuant to an exception or alternative granted under §201.26 or §610.68 of this chapter.

(ii) The applicant may distribute a product with a package insert, package label, or container label bearing such change at the time the change is made.

(4) *Advertisements and promotional labeling.* Advertisements and promotional labeling shall be submitted to the Center for Biologics Evaluation and Research or Center for Drug Evaluation and Research in accordance with the requirements set forth in §314.81(b)(3)(i) of this chapter.

(5) The submission and grant of a written request for an exception or alternative under §201.26 or §610.68 of this chapter satisfies the requirements in paragraphs (f)(1) through (f)(2) of this section.

(6) For purposes of paragraph (f)(2) of this section, information will be considered newly acquired if it consists of data, analyses, or other information not previously submitted to the agency, which may include (but are not limited to) data derived from new clinical studies, reports of adverse events, or new analyses of previously submitted data (e.g., meta-analyses) if the studies, events or analyses reveal risks of a different type or greater severity or frequency than previously included in submissions to FDA.

(g) *Failure to comply.* In addition to other remedies available in law and regulations, in the event of repeated failure of the applicant to comply with this section, FDA may require that the applicant submit a supplement for any proposed change and obtain approval of the supplement by FDA prior to distribution of the product made using the change.

(h) *Administrative review.* Under §10.75 of this chapter, an applicant may request internal FDA review of FDA employee decisions under this section.

[62 FR 39901, July 24, 1997, as amended at 63 FR 66399, Dec. 1, 1998. Redesignated at 65 FR 59718, Oct. 6, 2000, and amended at 69 FR 18766, Apr. 8, 2004; 70 FR 14983, Mar. 24, 2005; 71 FR 3997, Jan. 24, 2006; 72 FR 73600, Dec. 28, 2007; 73 FR 49609, Aug. 22, 2008; 73 FR 68333, Nov. 18, 2008; 80 FR 18092, Apr. 3, 2015]

§601.14   Regulatory submissions in electronic format.

(a) *General.* Electronic format submissions must be in a form that FDA can process, review, and archive. FDA will periodically issue guidance on how to provide the electronic submission (e.g., method of transmission, media, file formats, preparation and organization of files.)

(b) *Labeling.* The content of labeling required under §201.100(d)(3) of this chapter (commonly referred to as the package insert or professional labeling), including all text, tables, and figures, must be submitted to the agency in electronic format as described in paragraph (a) of this section. This requirement is in addition to the provisions of §§601.2(a) and 601.12(f) that require applicants to submit specimens of the labels, enclosures, and containers, or to submit other final printed labeling. Submissions under this paragraph must be made in accordance with part 11 of this chapter except for the requirements of §11.10(a), (c) through (h), and (k), and the corresponding requirements of §11.30.

[68 FR 69020, Dec. 11, 2003]

§601.15   Foreign establishments and products: samples for each importation.

Random samples of each importation, obtained by the District Director of Customs and forwarded to the Director, Center for Biologics Evaluation and Research or the Director, Center for Drug Evaluation and Research (see mailing addresses in §600.2(c) of this chapter) must be at least two final containers of each lot of product. A copy of the associated documents which describe and identify the shipment must accompany the shipment for forwarding with the samples to the Director, Center for Biologics Evaluation and Research or the Director, Center for Drug Evaluation and Research (see mailing addresses in §600.2(c)). For shipments of 20 or less final containers, samples need not be forwarded, provided a copy of an official release from the Center for Biologics Evaluation and Research or Center for Drug Evaluation and Research accompanies each shipment.

[70 FR 14983, Mar. 24, 2005, as amended at 80 FR 18092, Apr. 3, 2015]

§601.20   Biologics licenses; issuance and conditions.

(a) *Examination--compliance with requirements.* A biologics license application shall be approved only upon examination of the product and upon a determination that the product complies with the standards established in the biologics license application and the requirements prescribed in the regulations in this chapter including but not limited to the good manufacturing practice requirements set forth in parts 210, 211, 600, 606, and 820 of this chapter.

(b) *Availability of product.* No biologics license shall be issued unless:

(1) The product intended for introduction into interstate commerce is available for examination, and

(2) Such product is available for inspection during all phases of manufacture.

(c) *Manufacturing process—impairment of assurances.* No product shall be licensed if any part of the process of or relating to the manufacture of such product, in the judgment of the Director, Center for Biologics Evaluation and Research, would impair the assurances of continued safety, purity, and potency as provided by the regulations contained in this chapter.

(d) *Inspection—compliance with requirements.* A biologics license shall be issued or a biologics license application approved only after inspection of the establishment(s) listed in the biologics license application and upon a determination that the establishment(s) complies with the standards established in the biologics license application and the requirements prescribed in applicable regulations.

(e) *One biologics license to cover all locations.* One biologics license shall be issued to cover all locations meeting the establishment standards identified in the approved biologics license application and each location shall be subject to inspection by FDA officials.

[64 FR 56451, Oct. 20, 1999, as amended at 70 FR 14983, Mar. 24, 2005]

§601.21   Products under development.

A biological product undergoing development, but not yet ready for a biologics license, may be shipped or otherwise delivered from one State or possession into another State or possession provided such shipment or delivery is not for introduction or delivery for introduction into interstate commerce, except as provided in sections 505(i) and 520(g) of the Federal Food, Drug, and Cosmetic Act, as amended, and the regulations thereunder (21 CFR parts 312 and 812).

[64 FR 56451, Oct. 20, 1999]

§601.22   Products in short supply; initial manufacturing at other than licensed location.

A biologics license issued to a manufacturer and covering all locations of manufacture shall authorize persons other than such manufacturer to conduct at places other than such locations the initial, and partial manufacturing of a product for shipment solely to such manufacturer only to the extent that the names of such persons and places are registered with the Commissioner of Food and Drugs and it is found upon application of such manufacturer, that the product is in short supply due either to the peculiar growth requirements of the organism involved or to the scarcity of the animal required for manufacturing purposes, and such manufacturer has established with respect to such persons and places such procedures, inspections, tests or other arrangements as will ensure full compliance with the applicable regulations of this subchapter related to continued safety, purity, and potency. Such persons and places shall be subject to all regulations of this subchapter except §§601.2 to 601.6, 601.9, 601.10, 601.20, 601.21 to 601.33, and 610.60 to 610.65 of this chapter. For persons and places authorized under this section to conduct the

initial and partial manufacturing of a product for shipment solely to a manufacturer of a product subject to licensure under §601.2(c), the following additional regulations shall not be applicable: §§600.10(b) and (c), 600.11, 600.12, 600.13, and 610.53 of this chapter. Failure of such manufacturer to maintain such procedures, inspections, tests, or other arrangements, or failure of any person conducting such partial manufacturing to comply with applicable regulations shall constitute a ground for suspension or revocation of the authority conferred pursuant to this section on the same basis as provided in §§601.6 to 601.8 with respect to the suspension and the
revocation of licenses.

[42 FR 4718, Jan. 25, 1977, as amended at 61 FR 24233, May 14, 1996; 64 FR 56452, Oct. 20, 1999; 80 FR 37974, July 2, 2015]

§601.27   Pediatric studies.

(a) *Required assessment.* Except as provided in paragraphs (b), (c), and (d) of this section, each application for a new active ingredient, new indication, new dosage form, new dosing regimen, or new route of administration shall contain data that are adequate to assess the safety and effectiveness of the product for the claimed indications in all relevant pediatric subpopulations, and to support dosing and administration for each pediatric subpopulation for which the product is safe and effective. Where the course of the disease and the effects of the product are similar in adults and pediatric patients, FDA may conclude that pediatric effectiveness can be extrapolated from adequate and well-controlled effectiveness studies in adults, usually supplemented with other information in pediatric patients, such as pharmacokinetic studies. In addition, studies may not be needed in each pediatric age group, if data from one age group can be extrapolated to another. Assessments required under this section for a product that represents a meaningful therapeutic benefit over existing treatments must be carried out using appropriate formulations for the age group(s) for which the assessment is required.

(b) *Deferred submission*. (1) FDA may, on its own initiative or at the request of an applicant, defer submission of some or all assessments of safety and effectiveness described in paragraph (a) of this section until after licensing of the product for use in adults. Deferral may be granted if, among other reasons, the product is ready for approval in adults before studies in pediatric patients are complete, pediatric studies should be delayed until additional safety or effectiveness data have been collected. If an applicant requests deferred submission, the request must provide an adequate justification for delaying pediatric studies, a description of the planned or ongoing studies, and evidence that the studies are being or will be conducted with due diligence and at the earliest possible time.

(2) If FDA determines that there is an adequate justification for temporarily delaying the submission of assessments of pediatric safety and effectiveness, the product may be licensed for use in adults subject to the requirement that the applicant submit the required assessments within a specified time.

(c) *Waivers*—(1) *General*. FDA may grant a full or partial waiver of the requirements of paragraph (a) of this section on its own initiative or at the request of an applicant. A request for a waiver must provide an adequate justification.

(2) *Full waiver*. An applicant may request a waiver of the requirements of paragraph (a) of this section if the applicant certifies that:

(i) The product does not represent a meaningful therapeutic benefit over existing therapies for pediatric patients and is not likely to be used in a substantial number of pediatric patients;

(ii) Necessary studies are impossible or highly impractical because, e.g., the number of such patients is so small or geographically dispersed; or

(iii) There is evidence strongly suggesting that the product would be ineffective or unsafe in all pediatric age groups.

(3) *Partial waiver*. An applicant may request a waiver of the requirements of paragraph (a) of this section with respect to a specified pediatric age group, if the applicant certifies that:

(i) The product does not represent a meaningful therapeutic benefit over existing therapies for pediatric patients in that age group, and is not likely to be used in a substantial number of patients in that age group;

(ii) Necessary studies are impossible or highly impractical because, e.g., the number of patients in that age group is so small or geographically dispersed;

(iii) There is evidence strongly suggesting that the product would be ineffective or unsafe in that age group; or

(iv) The applicant can demonstrate that reasonable attempts to produce a pediatric formulation necessary for that age group have failed.

(4) *FDA action on waiver.* FDA shall grant a full or partial waiver, as appropriate, if the agency finds that there is a reasonable basis on which to conclude that one or more of the grounds for waiver specified in paragraphs (c)(2) or (c)(3) of this section have been met. If a waiver is granted on the ground that it is not possible to develop a pediatric formulation, the waiver will cover only those pediatric age groups requiring that formulation. If a waiver is granted because there is evidence that the product would be ineffective or unsafe in pediatric populations, this information will be included in the product's labeling.

(5) *Definition of "meaningful therapeutic benefit".* For purposes of this section, a product will be considered to offer a meaningful therapeutic benefit over existing therapies if FDA estimates that:

(i) If approved, the product would represent a significant improvement in the treatment, diagnosis, or prevention of a disease, compared to marketed products adequately labeled for that use in the relevant pediatric population. Examples of how improvement might be demonstrated include, e.g., evidence of increased effectiveness in treatment, prevention, or diagnosis of disease; elimination or substantial reduction of a treatment-limiting drug reaction; documented enhancement of compliance; or evidence of safety and effectiveness in a new subpopulation; or

(ii) The product is in a class of products or for an indication for which there is a need for additional therapeutic options.

(d) *Exemption for orphan drugs.* This section does not apply to any product for an indication or indications for which orphan designation has been granted under part 316, subpart C, of this chapter.

[63 FR 66671, Dec. 2, 1998]

§601.28 Annual reports of postmarketing pediatric studies.

Sponsors of licensed biological products shall submit the following information each year within 60 days of the anniversary date of approval of each product under the license to the Director, Center for Biologics Evaluation and Research or the Director, Center for Drug Evaluation and Research (see mailing addresses in §600.2(a) or (b) of this chapter):

(a) *Summary.* A brief summary stating whether labeling supplements for pediatric use have been submitted and whether new studies in the pediatric population to support appropriate labeling for the pediatric population have been initiated. Where possible, an estimate of patient exposure to the drug product, with special reference to the pediatric population (neonates, infants, children, and adolescents) shall be provided, including dosage form.

(b) *Clinical data.* Analysis of available safety and efficacy data in the pediatric population and changes proposed in the labeling based on this information. An assessment of data needed to ensure appropriate labeling for the pediatric population shall be included.

(c) *Status reports.* A statement on the current status of any postmarketing studies in the pediatric population performed by, or on behalf of, the applicant. The statement shall include whether postmarketing clinical studies in pediatric populations were required or agreed to, and, if so, the status of these studies shall be reported to FDA in annual progress reports of postmarketing studies under §601.70 rather than under this section.

[65 FR 59718, Oct. 6, 2000, as amended at 65 FR 64618, Oct. 30, 2000; 70 FR 14984, Mar. 24, 2005; 80 FR 18092, Apr. 3, 2015

§601.29　　Guidance documents.

(a) FDA has made available guidance documents under §10.115 of this chapter to help you comply with certain requirements of this part.

(b) The Center for Biologics Evaluation and Research (CBER) maintains a list of guidance documents that apply to the center's regulations. The lists are maintained on the Internet and are published annually in the Federal Register. You may request a copy of the CBER list from the Food and Drug Administration, Center for Biologics Evaluation and Research, Office of Communication, Outreach and Development, 10903 New Hampshire Ave., Bldg. 71, Rm. 3103, Silver Spring, MD 20993-0002.

[65 FR 56480, Sept. 19, 2000, as amended at 70 FR 14984, Mar. 24, 2005; 80 FR 18092, Apr. 3, 2015]

Subpart D--Diagnostic Radiopharmaceuticals

Source: 64 FR 26668, May 17, 1999, unless otherwise noted.

§601.30　　Scope.

This subpart applies to radiopharmaceuticals intended for in vivo administration for diagnostic and monitoring use. It does not apply to radiopharmaceuticals intended for therapeutic purposes. In situations where a particular radiopharmaceutical is proposed for both diagnostic and therapeutic uses, the radiopharmaceutical must be evaluated taking into account each intended use.

§601.31　　Definition.

For purposes of this part, *diagnostic radiopharmaceutical* means:

(a) An article that is intended for use in the diagnosis or monitoring of a disease or a manifestation of a disease in humans and that exhibits spontaneous disintegration of unstable nuclei with the emission of nuclear particles or photons; or

(b) Any nonradioactive reagent kit or nuclide generator that is intended to be used in the preparation of such article as defined in paragraph (a) of this section.

§601.32 General factors relevant to safety and effectiveness.

FDA's determination of the safety and effectiveness of a diagnostic radiopharmaceutical includes consideration of the following:

(a) The proposed use of the diagnostic radiopharmaceutical in the practice of medicine;

(b) The pharmacological and toxicological activity of the diagnostic radiopharmaceutical (including any carrier or ligand component of the diagnostic radiopharmaceutical); and

(c) The estimated absorbed radiation dose of the diagnostic radiopharmaceutical.

§601.33 Indications.

(a) For diagnostic radiopharmaceuticals, the categories of proposed indications for use include, but are not limited to, the following:

(1) Structure delineation;

(2) Functional, physiological, or biochemical assessment;

(3) Disease or pathology detection or assessment; and

(4) Diagnostic or therapeutic patient management.

(b) Where a diagnostic radiopharmaceutical is not intended to provide disease-specific information, the proposed indications for use may refer to a biochemical, physiological, anatomical, or pathological process or to more than one disease or condition.

§601.34 Evaluation of effectiveness.

(a) The effectiveness of a diagnostic radiopharmaceutical is assessed by evaluating its ability to provide useful clinical information related to its proposed indications for use. The method of this evaluation varies depending upon the proposed indication(s) and may use one or more of the following criteria:

(1) The claim of structure delineation is established by demonstrating in a defined clinical setting the ability to locate anatomical structures and to characterize their anatomy.

(2) The claim of functional, physiological, or biochemical

assessment is established by demonstrating in a defined clinical setting reliable measurement of function(s) or physiological, biochemical, or molecular process(es).

(3) The claim of disease or pathology detection or assessment is established by demonstrating in a defined clinical setting that the diagnostic radiopharmaceutical has sufficient accuracy in identifying or characterizing the disease or pathology.

(4) The claim of diagnostic or therapeutic patient management is established by demonstrating in a defined clinical setting that the test is useful in diagnostic or therapeutic patient management.

(5) For a claim that does not fall within the indication categories identified in §601.33, the applicant or sponsor should consult FDA on how to establish the effectiveness of the diagnostic radiopharmaceutical for the claim.

(b) The accuracy and usefulness of the diagnostic information is determined by comparison with a reliable assessment of actual clinical status. A reliable assessment of actual clinical status may be provided by a diagnostic standard or standards of demonstrated accuracy. In the absence of such diagnostic standard(s), the actual clinical status must be established in another manner, e.g., patient followup.

§601.35   Evaluation of safety.

(a) Factors considered in the safety assessment of a diagnostic radiopharmaceutical include, among others, the following:

(1) The radiation dose;

(2) The pharmacology and toxicology of the radiopharmaceutical, including any radionuclide, carrier, or ligand;

(3) The risks of an incorrect diagnostic determination;

(4) The adverse reaction profile of the drug;

(5) Results of human experience with the radiopharmaceutical for other uses; and

(6) Results of any previous human experience with the carrier or ligand of the radiopharmaceutical when the same chemical entity as the carrier or ligand has been used in a previously studied product.

(b) The assessment of the adverse reaction profile includes, but is not limited to, an evaluation of the potential of the diagnostic radiopharmaceutical, including the carrier or ligand, to elicit the following:

(1) Allergic or hypersensitivity responses,

(2) Immunologic responses,

(3) Changes in the physiologic or biochemical function of the target and nontarget tissues, and

(4) Clinically detectable signs or symptoms.

(c)(1) To establish the safety of a diagnostic radiopharmaceutical, FDA may require, among other information, the following types of data:

(A) Pharmacology data,

(B) Toxicology data,

(C) Clinical adverse event data, and

(D) Radiation safety assessment.

(2) The amount of new safety data required will depend on the characteristics of the product and available information regarding the safety of the diagnostic radiopharmaceutical, and its carrier or ligand, obtained from other studies and uses. Such information may include, but is not limited to, the dose, route of administration, frequency of use, half-life of the ligand or carrier, half-life of the radionuclide, and results of clinical and preclinical studies. FDA will establish categories of diagnostic radiopharmaceuticals based on defined characteristics relevant to risk and will specify the amount and type of safety data that are appropriate for each category (e.g., required safety data may be limited for diagnostic radiopharmaceuticals with a well established, low-risk profile). Upon reviewing the relevant product characteristics and safety information, FDA will place each diagnostic radiopharmaceutical into the appropriate safety risk category.

(d) *Radiation safety assessment.* The radiation safety assessment must establish the radiation dose of a diagnostic radiopharmaceutical by radiation dosimetry evaluations in humans and appropriate animal models. The maximum tolerated dose need not be established.

Subpart E-- Accelerated Approval of Biological Products for Serious or Life-Threatening Illnesses

Source: 57 FR 58959, Dec. 11, 1992, unless otherwise noted.

§601.40   Scope.

This subpart applies to certain biological products that have been studied for their safety and effectiveness in treating serious or life-threatening illnesses and that provide meaningful therapeutic benefit to patients over existing treatments (e.g., ability to treat patients unresponsive to, or intolerant of, available therapy, or improved patient response over available therapy).

§601.41   Approval based on a surrogate endpoint or on an effect on a clinical endpoint other than survival or irreversible morbidity.

FDA may grant marketing approval for a biological product on the basis of adequate and well-controlled clinical trials establishing that the biological product has an effect on a surrogate endpoint that is reasonably likely, based on epidemiologic, therapeutic, pathophysiologic, or other evidence, to predict clinical benefit or on the basis of an effect on a clinical endpoint other than survival or irreversible morbidity. Approval under this section will be subject to the requirement that the applicant study the biological product further, to verify and describe its clinical benefit, where there is uncertainty as to the relation of the surrogate endpoint to clinical benefit, or of the observed clinical benefit to ultimate outcome. Postmarketing studies would usually be studies already underway. When required to be conducted, such studies must also be adequate and well-controlled. The applicant shall carry out any such studies with due diligence.

§601.42   Approval with restrictions to assure safe use.

(a) If FDA concludes that a biological product shown to be effective can be safely used only if distribution or use is restricted, FDA will require such postmarketing restrictions as are needed to assure safe use of the biological product, such as:

(1) Distribution restricted to certain facilities or physicians with special training or experience; or

(2) Distribution conditioned on the performance of specified medical procedures.

(b) The limitations imposed will be commensurate with the specific safety concerns presented by the biological product.

§601.43   Withdrawal procedures.

(a) For biological products approved under §601.41or §601.42, FDA may withdraw approval, following a hearing as provided in part 15 of this chapter, as modified by this section, if:

(1) A postmarketing clinical study fails to verify clinical benefit;

(2) The applicant fails to perform the required postmarketing study with due diligence;

(3) Use after marketing demonstrates that postmarketing restrictions are inadequate to ensure safe use of the biological product;

(4) The applicant fails to adhere to the postmarketing restrictions agreed upon;

(5) The promotional materials are false or misleading; or

(6) Other evidence demonstrates that the biological product is not shown to be safe or effective under its conditions of use.

(b) *Notice of opportunity for a hearing.* The Director of the Center for Biologics Evaluation and Research will give the applicant notice of an opportunity for a hearing on the Center's proposal to withdraw the approval of an application approved under §601.41 or §601.42. The notice, which will ordinarily be a letter, will state generally the reasons for the action and the proposed grounds for the order.

(c) *Submission of data and information.* (1) If the applicant fails to file a written request for a hearing within 15 days of receipt of the notice, the applicant waives the opportunity for a hearing.

(2) If the applicant files a timely request for a hearing, the agency will publish a notice of hearing in the FEDERAL REGISTER in accordance with §12.32(e) and 15.20 of this chapter.

(3) An applicant who requests a hearing under this section must, within 30 days of receipt of the notice of opportunity for a hearing, submit the data and information upon which the applicant intends to rely at the hearing.

(d) *Separation of functions.* Separation of functions (as specified in §10.55 of this chapter) will not apply at any point in withdrawal proceedings under this section.

(e) *Procedures for hearings.* Hearings held under this section will be conducted in accordance with the provisions of part 15 of this chapter, with the following modifications:

(1) An advisory committee duly constituted under part 14 of this chapter will be present at the hearing. The committee will be asked to review the issues involved and to provide advice and recommendations to the Commissioner of Food and Drugs.

(2) The presiding officer, the advisory committee members, up to three representatives of the applicant, and up to three representatives of the Center may question any person during or at the conclusion of the person's presentation. No other person attending the hearing may question a person making a presentation. The presiding officer may, as a matter of discretion, permit questions to be submitted to the presiding officer for response by a person making a presentation.

(f) *Judicial review.* The Commissioner's decision constitutes final agency action from which the applicant may petition for judicial review. Before requesting an order from a court for a stay of action pending review, an applicant must first submit a petition for a stay of action under §10.35 of this chapter.

[57 FR 58959, Dec. 11, 1992, as amended at 68 FR 34797, June 11, 2003; 70 FR 14984, Mar. 24, 2005]

§601.44 Postmarketing safety reporting.

Biological products approved under this program are subject to the postmarketing recordkeeping and safety reporting applicable to all approved biological products.

§601.45 Promotional materials.

For biological products being considered for approval under this subpart, unless otherwise informed by the agency, applicants must submit to the agency for consideration during the preapproval review period copies of all promotional materials, including promotional labeling as well as advertisements, intended for dissemination or publication within 120 days following marketing approval. After 120 days following marketing approval, unless otherwise informed by the agency, the applicant must submit promotional materials at least 30 days prior to the intended time of initial dissemination of the labeling or initial publication of the advertisement

§601.46 Termination of requirements.

If FDA determines after approval that the requirements established in §601.42, §601.43, or §601.45 are no longer necessary for the safe and effective use of a biological product, it will so notify the applicant. Ordinarily, for biological products approved under §601.41, these requirements will no longer apply when FDA determines that the required postmarketing study verifies and describes the biological product's clinical benefit and the biological product would be appropriate for approval under traditional procedures. For biological products approved under §601.42, the restrictions would no longer apply when FDA determines that safe use of the biological product can be assured through appropriate labeling. FDA also retains the discretion to remove specific postapproval requirements upon review of a petition submitted by the sponsor in accordance with §10.30.

Subpart F--Confidentiality of Information

§601.50 Confidentiality of data and information in an investigational new drug notice for a biological product.

(a) The existence of an IND notice for a biological product will not be disclosed by the Food and Drug Administration unless it has previously been publicly disclosed or acknowledged.

(b) The availability for public disclosure of all data and information in an IND file for a biological product shall be handled in accordance with the provisions established in §601.51.

(c) Notwithstanding the provisions of §601.51, the Food and Drug Administration shall disclose upon request to an individual on whom an investigational biological product has been used a copy of any adverse reaction report relating to such use.

[39 FR 44656, Dec. 24, 1974]

§601.51 Confidentiality of data and information in applications for biologics licenses.

(a) For purposes of this section the biological product file includes all data and information submitted with or incorporated by reference in any application for a biologics license, IND's incorporated into any such application, master files, and other related submissions. The availability for public disclosure of any record in the biological product file shall be handled in accordance with the provisions of this section.

(b) The existence of a biological product file will not be disclosed by the Food and Drug Administration before a biologics license application has been approved unless it has previously been publicly disclosed or acknowledged. The Director of the Center for Biologics Evaluation and Research will maintain a list available for public disclosure of biological products for which a license application has been approved.

(c) If the existence of a biological product file has not been publicly disclosed or acknowledged, no data or information in the biological product file is available for public disclosure.

(d)(1) If the existence of a biological product file has been publicly disclosed or acknowledged before a license has been issued, no data or information contained in the file is available for public disclosure before such license is issued, but the Commissioner may, in his discretion, disclose a summary of such selected portions of the safety and effectiveness data as are appropriate for public consideration of a specific pending issue, e.g., at an open session of a Food and Drug Administration advisory committee or pursuant to an exchange of important regulatory information with a foreign government.

(2) Notwithstanding paragraph (d)(1) of this section, FDA will make available to the public upon request the information in the IND that was required to be filed in Docket Number 95S-0158 in the Dockets Management Branch (HFA-305), Food and Drug Administration, 5630 Fishers Lane, rm. 1061, Rockville, MD 20852, for investigations involving an exception from informed consent under § 50.24 of this chapter. Persons wishing to request this information shall submit a request under the Freedom of Information Act.

(e) After a license has been issued, the following data and information in the biological product file are immediately available for public disclosure unless extraordinary circumstances are shown:

(1) All safety and effectiveness data and information.

(2) A protocol for a test or study, unless it is shown to fall within the exemption established for trade secrets and confidential commercial or financial information in §20.61 of this chapter.

(3) Adverse reaction reports, product experience reports, consumer complaints, and other similar data and information, after deletion of:

(i) Names and any information that would identify the person using the product.

(ii) Names and any information that would identify any third party involved with the report, such as a physician or hospital or other institution.

(4) A list of all active ingredients and any inactive ingredients previously disclosed to the public, as defined in §20.81 of this chapter.

(5) An assay method or other analytical method, unless it serves no regulatory or compliance purpose and it is shown to fall within the exemption established in §20.61 of this chapter.

(6) All correspondence and written summaries of oral discussions relating to the biological product file, in accordance with the provisions of part 20 of this chapter.

(7) All records showing the manufacturer's testing of a particular lot, after deletion of data or information that would show the volume of the drug produced, manufacturing procedures and controls, yield from raw materials, costs, or other material falling within §20.61 of this chapter.

(8) All records showing the testing of and action on a particular lot by the Food and Drug Administration.

(f) The following data and information in a biological product file are not available for public disclosure unless they have been previously disclosed to the public as defined in §20.81 of this chapter or they relate to a product or ingredient that has been abandoned and they no longer represent a trade secret or confidential commercial or financial information as defined in §20.61 of this chapter:

(1) Manufacturing methods or processes, including quality control procedures.

(2) Production, sales, distribution, and similar data and information, except that any compilation of such data and information aggregated and prepared in a way that does not reveal data or information which is not available for public disclosure under this provision is available for public disclosure.

(3) Quantitative or semiquantitative formulas.

(g) For purposes of this regulation, safety and effectiveness data include all studies and tests of a biological product on animals and humans and all studies and tests on the drug for identity, stability, purity, potency, and bioavailability.

[39 FR 44656, Dec. 24, 1974, as amended at 42 FR 15676, Mar. 22, 1977; 49 FR 23833, June 8, 1984; 55 FR 11013, Mar. 26, 1990; 61 FR 51530, Oct. 2, 1996; 64 FR 56452, Oct. 20, 1999; 68 FR 24879, May 9, 2003; 69 FR 13717, Mar. 24, 2004; 70 FR 14984, Mar. 24, 2005]

Subpart G--Postmarketing Studies

Source: 65 FR 64618, Oct. 30, 2000, unless otherwise noted.

§601.70   Annual progress reports of post marketing studies.

(a) *General requirements*. This section applies to all required postmarketing studies (e.g., accelerated approval clinical benefit studies, pediatric studies) and postmarketing studies that an applicant has committed, in writing, to conduct either at the time of approval of an application or a supplement to an application, or after approval of an application or a supplement. Postmarketing studies within the meaning of this section are those that concern:

(1) Clinical safety;

(2) Clinical efficacy;

(3) Clinical pharmacology; and

(4) Nonclinical toxicology.

(b) *What to report*. Each applicant of a licensed biological product shall submit a report to FDA on the status of postmarketing studies for each approved product application. The status of these postmarketing studies shall be reported annually until FDA notifies the applicant, in writing, that the agency concurs with the applicant's determination that the study commitment has been fulfilled, or that the study is either no longer feasible or would no longer provide useful information. Each annual progress report shall be accompanied by a completed transmittal Form FDA-2252, and shall include all the information required under this section that the applicant received or otherwise obtained during the annual reporting interval which ends on the U.S. anniversary date. The report must provide the following information for each postmarketing study:

(1) *Applicant's name*.

(2) *Product name*. Include the approved product's proper name and the proprietary name, if any.

(3) *Biologics license application (BLA) and supplement number*.

(4) *Date of U.S. approval of BLA*.

(5) *Date of postmarketing study commitment*.

(6) *Description of postmarketing study commitment*.

The description must include sufficient information to uniquely describe the study. This information may include the purpose of the study, the type of study, the patient population addressed by the study and the indication(s) and dosage(s) that are to be studied.

(7) *Schedule for completion and reporting of the postmarketing study commitment.* The schedule should include the actual or projected dates for submission of the study protocol to FDA, completion of patient accrual or initiation of an animal study, completion of the study, submission of the final study report to FDA, and any additional milestones or submissions for which projected dates were specified as part of the commitment. In addition, it should include a revised schedule, as appropriate. If the schedule has been previously revised, provide both the original schedule and the most recent, previously submitted revision.

(8) *Current status of the postmarketing study commitment.* The status of each postmarketing study should be categorized using one of the following terms that describes the study's status on the anniversary date of U.S. approval of the application or other agreed upon date:

(i) *Pending.* The study has not been initiated, but does not meet the criterion for delayed.

(ii) *Ongoing.* The study is proceeding according to or ahead of the original schedule described under paragraph (b)(7) of this section.

(iii) *Delayed.* The study is behind the original schedule described under paragraph (b)(7) of this section.

(iv) *Terminated.* The study was ended before completion but a final study report has not been submitted to FDA.

(v) *Submitted.* The study has been completed or terminated and a final study report has been submitted to FDA.

(9) *Explanation of the study's status.* Provide a brief description of the status of the study, including the patient accrual rate (expressed by providing the number of patients or subjects enrolled to date, and the total planned enrollment), and an explanation of the study's status identified under paragraph (b)(8) of this section. If the study has been completed, include the date the study was completed and the date the final study report was submitted to FDA, as applicable. Provide a revised schedule, as well as the rea-

son(s) for the revision, if the schedule under paragraph (b)(7) of this section has changed since the previous report.

(c) *When to report.* Annual progress reports for postmarketing study commitments entered into by applicants shall be reported to FDA within 60 days of the anniversary date of the U.S. approval of the application for the product.

(d) *Where to report.* Submit two copies of the annual progress report of postmarketing studies to the Center for Biologics Evaluation and Research or Center for Drug Evaluation and Research (see mailing addresses in §600.2(a) or (b) of this chapter).

(e) *Public disclosure of information.* Except for the information described in this paragraph, FDA may publicly disclose any information concerning a postmarketing study, within the meaning of this section, if the agency determines that the information is necessary to identify an applicant or to establish the status of the study including the reasons, if any, for failure to conduct, complete, and report the study. Under this section, FDA will not publicly disclose trade secrets, as defined in §20.61 of this chapter, or information, described in §20.63 of this chapter, the disclosure of which would constitute an unwarranted invasion of personal privacy.

[65 FR 64618, Oct. 30, 2000, as amended at 70 FR 14984, Mar. 24, 2005; 80 FR 18092, Apr. 3, 2015]

Subpart H -- Approval of Biological Products When Human Efficacy Studies Are Not Ethical or Feasible

SOURCE: 67 FR 37996, May 31, 2002, unless otherwise noted.

§601.90   Scope.

This subpart applies to certain biological products that have been studied for their safety and efficacy in ameliorating or preventing serious or life-threatening conditions caused by exposure to lethal or permanently disabling toxic biological, chemical, radiological, or nuclear substances. This subpart applies only to those biological products for which: Definitive human efficacy studies cannot be conducted because it would be unethical to deliberately expose healthy human volunteers to a lethal or permanently disabling toxic biological, chemical, radiological, or nuclear substance; and field trials to study the product's efficacy after an accidental or hostile exposure have not been feasible. This subpart does not apply to products that can be approved based on efficacy standards described elsewhere in FDA's regulations (e.g., accelerated approval based on surrogate markers or clinical endpoints other than survival or irreversible morbidity), nor does it address the safety evaluation for the products to which it does apply.

§601.91 Approval based on evidence of effectiveness from studies in animals.

(a) FDA may grant marketing approval for a biological product for which safety has been established and for which the requirements of §601.90 are met based on adequate and well-controlled animal studies when the results of those animal studies establish that the biological product is reasonably likely to produce clinical benefit in humans. In assessing the sufficiency of animal data, the agency may take into account other data, including human data, available to the agency. FDA will rely on the evidence from studies in animals to provide substantial evidence of the effectiveness of these products only when:

(1) There is a reasonably well-understood pathophysiological mechanism of the toxicity of the substance and its prevention or substantial reduction by the product;

(2) The effect is demonstrated in more than one animal species expected to react with a response predictive for humans, unless the effect is demonstrated in a single animal species that represents a sufficiently well-characterized animal model for predicting the response in humans;

(3) The animal study endpoint is clearly related to the desired benefit in humans, generally the enhancement of survival or prevention of major morbidity; and

(4) The data or information on the kinetics and pharmacodynamics of the product or other relevant data or information, in animals and humans, allows selection of an effective dose in humans.

(b) Approval under this subpart will be subject to three requirements:

(1) *Postmarketing studies.* The applicant must conduct

postmarketing studies, such as field studies, to verify and describe the biological product's clinical benefit and to assess its safety when used as indicated when such studies are feasible and ethical. Such postmarketing studies would not be feasible until an exigency arises. When such studies are feasible, the applicant must conduct such studies with due diligence. Applicants must include as part of their application a plan or approach to postmarketing study commitments in the event such studies become ethical and feasible.

(2) *Approval with restrictions to ensure safe use.* If FDA concludes that a biological product shown to be effective under this subpart can be safely used only if distribution or use is restricted, FDA will require such postmarketing restrictions as are needed to ensure safe use of the biological product, commensurate with the specific safety concerns presented by the biological product, such as:

(i) Distribution restricted to certain facilities or health care practitioners with special training or experience;

(ii) Distribution conditioned on the performance of specified medical procedures, including medical followup; and

(iii) Distribution conditioned on specified recordkeeping requirements.

(3) *Information to be provided to patient recipients.* For biological products or specific indications approved under this subpart, applicants must prepare, as part of their proposed labeling, labeling to be provided to patient recipients. The patient labeling must explain that, for ethical or feasibility reasons, the biological product's approval was based on efficacy studies conducted in animals alone and must give the biological product's indication(s), directions for use (dosage and administration), contraindications, a description of any reasonably foreseeable risks, adverse reactions, anticipated benefits, drug interactions, and any other relevant information required by FDA at the time of approval. The patient labeling must be available with the product to be provided to patients prior to administration or dispensing of the biological product for the use approved under this subpart, if possible.

§601.92   Withdrawal procedures.

(a) *Reasons to withdraw approval.* For biological products approved under this subpart, FDA may withdraw approval, following a hearing as provided in part 15 of this chapter, as modified by this section, if:

(1) A postmarketing clinical study fails to verify clinical benefit;

(2) The applicant fails to perform the postmarketing study with due diligence;

(3) Use after marketing demonstrates that postmarketing restrictions are inadequate to ensure safe use of the biological product;

(4) The applicant fails to adhere to the postmarketing restrictions applied at the time of approval under this subpart;

(5) The promotional materials are false or misleading; or

(6) Other evidence demonstrates that the biological product is not shown to be safe or effective under its conditions of use.

(b) *Notice of opportunity for a hearing.* The Director of the Center for Biologics Evaluation and Research (CBER) will give the applicant notice of an opportunity for a hearing on CBER's proposal to withdraw the approval of an application approved under this subpart. The notice, which will ordinarily be a letter, will state generally the reasons for the action and the proposed grounds for the order.

(c) *Submission of data and information.* (1) If the applicant fails to file a written request for a hearing within 15 days of receipt of the notice, the applicant waives the opportunity for a hearing.

(2) If the applicant files a timely request for a hearing, the agency will publish a notice of hearing in the FEDERAL REGISTER in accordance with §§12.32(e) and 15.20 of this chapter.

(3) An applicant who requests a hearing under this section must, within 30 days of receipt of the notice of opportunity for a hearing, submit the data and information upon which the applicant intends to rely at the hearing.

(d) *Separation of functions.* Separation of functions (as specified in §10.55 of this chapter) will not apply at any point in withdrawal proceedings under this section.

(e) *Procedures for hearings*. Hearings held under this section will be conducted in accordance with the provisions of part 15 of this chapter, with the following modifications:

(1) An advisory committee duly constituted under part 14 of this chapter will be present at the hearing. The committee will be asked to review the issues involved and to provide advice and recommendations to the Commissioner of Food and Drugs.

(2) The presiding officer, the advisory committee members, up to three representatives of the applicant, and up to three representatives of CBER may question any person during or at the conclusion of the person's presentation. No other person attending the hearing may question a person making a presentation. The presiding officer may, as a matter of discretion, permit questions to be submitted to the presiding officer for response by a person making a presentation.

(f) *Judicial review*. The Commissioner of Food and Drugs' decision constitutes final agency action from which the applicant may petition for judicial review. Before requesting an order from a court for a stay of action pending review, an applicant must first submit a petition for a stay of action under §10.35 of this chapter.

[67 FR 37996, May 31, 2002, as amended at 70 FR 14984, Mar. 24, 2005]

§601.93   Postmarketing safety reporting.

Biological products approved under this subpart are subject to the postmarketing recordkeeping and safety reporting applicable to all approved biological products.

§601.94   Promotional materials.

For biological products being considered for approval under this subpart, unless otherwise informed by the agency, applicants must submit to the agency for consideration during the preapproval review period copies of all promotional materials, including promotional labeling as well as advertisements, intended for dissemination or publication within 120 days following marketing approval. After 120 days following marketing approval, unless otherwise informed by the agency, the applicant must submit promotional materials at least 30 days prior to the intended time of initial dissemination of the labeling or initial publication of the advertisement.

§601.95   Termination of requirements.

If FDA determines after approval under this subpart that the requirements established in §§601.91(b)(2), 601.92, and 601.93 are no longer necessary for the safe and effective use of a biological product, FDA will so notify the applicant. Ordinarily, for biological products approved under §601.91, these requirements will no longer apply when FDA determines that the postmarketing study verifies and describes the biological product's clinical benefit. For biological products approved under §601.91, the restrictions would no longer apply when FDA determines that safe use of the biological product can be ensured through appropriate labeling. FDA also retains the discretion to remove specific postapproval requirements upon review of a petition submitted by the sponsor in accordance with §10.30 of this chapter.

Notes

Notes

The Code of Federal Regulations
Title 21 – Food and Drugs

Part 610
GENERAL BIOLOGICAL
PRODUCTS STANDARDS

Printed by GMP Publications, Inc.
Tel: 866-544-9007 or 856-810-7331
Fax: 866-544-9002
http://www.gmppublications.com
sales@gmppublications.com

PART 610-- GENERAL BIOLOGICAL PRODUCTS STANDARDS

Subpart F--Dating Period Limitations

§610.50   Date of manufacture for biological products.
§610.53   Dating periods for Whole Blood and blood components.

Subpart G--Labeling Standards

§610.60   Container label.
§610.61   Package label.
§610.62   Proper name; package label; legible type.
§610.63   Divided manufacturing responsibility to be shown.
§610.64   Name and address of distributor.
§610.65   Products for export.
§610.67   Bar code label requirements.
§610.68   Exceptions or alternatives to labeling requirements for biological products held by the Strategic National Stockpile.

Authority: 21 U.S.C. 321, 331, 351, 352, 353, 355, 360, 360c, 360d, 360h, 360i, 371, 372, 374, 381; 42 U.S.C. 216, 262, 263, 263a, 264.

Source: 38 FR 32056, Nov. 20, 1973, unless otherwise noted.

Cross References: For U.S. Customs Service regulations relating to viruses, serums, and toxins, see 19 CFR 12.21--12.23. For U.S. Postal Service regulations relating to the admissibility to the United States mails see parts 124 and 125 of the Domestic Mail Manual, that is incorporated by reference in 39 CFR part 111.

Subpart A--Release Requirements

§610.1   Tests prior to release required for each lot.

No lot of any licensed product shall be released by the manufacturer prior to the completion of tests for conformity with standards applicable to such product. Each applicable test shall be made on each lot after completion of all processes of manufacture which may affect compliance with the standard to which the test applies. The results of all tests performed shall be considered in determining whether or not the test results meet the test objective, except that a test result may be disregarded when it is established that the test is invalid due to causes unrelated to the product.

§610.2   Requests for samples and protocols; official release.

(a) *Licensed biological products regulated by CBER.* Samples of any lot of any licensed product together with the protocols showing results of applicable tests, may at any time be required to be sent to the Director, Center for Biologics Evaluation and Research (see mailing addresses in §600.2(c) of this chapter). Upon notification by the Director, Center for Biologics Evaluation and Research, a manufacturer shall not distribute a lot of a product until the lot is released by the Director, Center for Biologics Evaluation and Research: Provided, That the Director, Center for Biologics Evaluation and Research, shall not issue such notification except when deemed necessary for the safety, purity, or potency of the product.

(b) *Licensed biological products regulated by CDER.* Samples of any lot of any licensed product together with the protocols showing results of applicable tests, may at any time be required to be sent to the Director, Center for Drug Evaluation and Research (see mailing addresses in §600.2(c) of this chapter) for official release. Upon notification by the Director, Center for Drug Evaluation and

Research, a manufacturer shall not distribute a lot of a biological product until the lot is released by the Director, Center for Drug Evaluation and Research: Provided, That the Director, Center for Drug Evaluation and Research shall not issue such notification except when deemed necessary for the safety, purity, or potency of the product.

[40 FR 31313, July 25, 1975, as amended at 49 FR 23834, June 8, 1984; 50 FR 10941, Mar. 19, 1985; 55 FR 11013 and 11014, Mar. 26, 1990; 67 FR 9587, Mar. 4, 2002; 70 FR 14984, Mar. 24, 2005; 80 FR 18093, Apr. 3, 2015]

Subpart B--General Provisions

§610.9   Equivalent methods and processes.

Modification of any particular test method or manufacturing process or the conditions under which it is conducted as required in this part or in the additional standards for specific biological products in parts 620 through 680 of this chapter shall be permitted only under the following conditions:

(a) The applicant presents evidence, in the form of a license application, or a supplement to the application submitted in accordance with §601.12(b) or (c), demonstrating that the modification will provide assurances of the safety, purity, potency, and effectiveness of the biological product equal to or greater than the assurances provided by the method or process specified in the general standards or additional standards for the biological product; and

(b) Approval of the modification is received in writing from the Director, Center for Biologics Evaluation and Research, or the Director, Center for Drug Evaluation and Research.

[62 FR 39903, July 24, 1997, as amended at 70 FR 14984, Mar. 24, 2005]

§610.10   Potency.

Tests for potency shall consist of either in vitro or in vivo tests, or both, which have been specifically designed for each product so as to indicate its potency in a manner adequate to satisfy the interpretation of potency given by the definition in §600.3(s) of this chapter.

§610.11-610.11a [Reserved]

§610.12 Sterility.

(a) *The test.* Except as provided in paragraph (h) of this section, manufacturers of biological products must perform sterility testing of each lot of each biological product's final container material or other material, as appropriate and as approved in the biologics license application or supplement for that product.

(b) *Test requirements.* (1) The sterility test must be appropriate to the material being tested such that the material does not interfere with or otherwise hinder the test.

(2) The sterility test must be validated to demonstrate that the test is capable of reliably and consistently detecting the presence of viable contaminating microorganisms.

(3) The sterility test and test components must be verified to demonstrate that the test method can consistently detect the presence of viable contaminating microorganisms.

(c) *Written procedures.* Manufacturers must establish, implement, and follow written procedures for sterility testing that describe, at a minimum, the following:

(1) The sterility test method to be used;

(i) If culture-based test methods are used, include, at a minimum:

(A) Composition of the culture media;

(B) Growth-promotion test requirements; and

(C) Incubation conditions (time and temperature).

(ii) If non-culture-based test methods are used, include, at a minimum:

(A) Composition of test components;

(B) Test parameters, including acceptance criteria; and

(C) Controls used to verify the method's ability to detect the presence of viable contaminating microorganisms.

(2) The method of sampling, including the number, volume, and size of articles to be tested;

(3) Written specifications for the acceptance or rejection of each lot; and

(4) A statement of any other function critical to the particular sterility test method to ensure consistent and accurate results.

(d) *The sample.* The sample must be appropriate to the material being tested, considering, at a minimum:

(1) The size and volume of the final product lot;

(2) The duration of manufacturing of the drug product;

(3) The final container configuration and size;

(4) The quantity or concentration of inhibitors, neutralizers, and preservatives, if present, in the tested material;

(5) For a culture-based test method, the volume of test material that results in a dilution of the product that is not bacteriostatic or fungistatic; and

(6) For a non-culture-based test method, the volume of test material that results in a dilution of the product that does not inhibit or otherwise hinder the detection of viable contaminating microorganisms.

(e) *Verification.* (1) For culture-based test methods, studies must be conducted to demonstrate that the performance of the test organisms and culture media are suitable to consistently detect the presence of viable contaminating microorganisms, including tests for each lot of culture media to verify its growth- promoting properties over the shelf-life of the media.

(2) For non-culture-based test methods, within the test itself, appropriate controls must be used to demonstrate the ability of the test method to continue to consistently detect the presence of viable contaminating microorganisms.

(f) *Repeat test procedures.-* (1) If the initial test indicates the presence of microorganisms, the product does not comply with the sterility test requirements unless a thorough investigation by the quality control unit can ascribe definitively the microbial presence to a laboratory error or faulty materials used in conducting the sterility testing.

(2) If the investigation described in paragraph (f)(1) of this section finds that the initial test indicated the presence of microorganisms due to laboratory error or the use of faulty materials, a sterility test may be repeated one time.

If no evidence of microorganisms is found in the repeat test, the product examined complies with the sterility test requirements. If evidence of microorganisms is found in the repeat test, the product examined does not comply with the sterility test requirements.

(3) If a repeat test is conducted, the same test method must be used for both the initial and repeat tests, and the repeat test must be conducted with comparable product that is reflective of the initial sample in terms of sample location and the stage in the manufacturing process from which it was obtained.

(g) *Records*. The records related to the test requirements of this section must be prepared and maintained as required by §§ 211.167 and 211.194 of this chapter.

(h) *Exceptions*. Sterility testing must be performed on final container material or other appropriate material as defined in the approved biologics license application or supplement and as described in this section, except as follows:

(1) This section does not require sterility testing for Whole Blood, Cryoprecipitated Antihemophilic Factor, Platelets, Red Blood Cells, Plasma, Source Plasma, Smallpox Vaccine, Reagent Red Blood Cells, Anti- Human Globulin, and Blood Grouping Reagents.

(2) A manufacturer is not required to comply with the sterility test requirements if the Director of the Center for Biologics Evaluation and Research or the Director of the Center for Drug Evaluation and Research, as appropriate, determines that data submitted in the biologics license application or supplement adequately establish that the route of administration, the method of preparation, or any other aspect of the product precludes or does not necessitate a sterility test to assure the safety, purity, and potency of the product. [77 FR 26174, May 3, 2012]

§610.13   Purity.

Products shall be free of extraneous material except that which is unavoidable in the manufacturing process described in the approved biologics license application. In addition, products shall be tested as provided in paragraphs (a) and (b) of this section.

(a)(1) *Test for residual moisture*. Each lot of dried product shall be tested for residual moisture and shall meet and not exceed established limits as specified by an approved method on file in the biologics license application. The test for residual moisture may be exempted by the Director, Center for Biologics Evaluation and Research or the Director, Center for Drug Evaluation and Research when deemed not necessary for the continued safety, purity, and potency of the product.

(2) *Records*. Appropriate records for residual moisture under paragraph (a)(1) of this section shall be prepared and maintained as required by the applicable provisions of § 211.188 and 211.194 of this chapter.

(b) *Test for pyrogenic substances*. Each lot of final containers of any product intended for use by injection shall be tested for pyrogenic substances by intravenous injection into rabbits as provided in paragraphs (b) (1) and (2) of this section: *Provided*, That notwithstanding any other provision of Subchapter F of this chapter, the test for pyrogenic substances is not required for the following products: Products containing formed blood elements; Cryopreci-pitate; Plasma; Source Plasma; Normal Horse Serum; bacterial, viral, and rickettsial vaccines and antigens; toxoids; toxins; allergenic extracts; venoms; diagnostic substances and trivalent organic arsenicals.

(1) *Test dose*. The test dose for each rabbit shall be at least 3 milliliters per kilogram of body weight of the rabbit and also shall be at least equivalent proportionately, on a body weight basis, to the maximum single human dose recommended, but need not exceed 10 milliliters per kilogram of body weight of the rabbit, except that: (i) Regardless of the human dose recommended, the test

dose per kilogram of body weight of each rabbit shall be at least 1 milliliter for immune globulins derived from human blood; (ii) for Streptokinase, the test dose shall be at least equivalent proportionately, on a body weight basis, to the maximum single human dose recommended.

(2) *Test procedure, results, and interpretation; standards to be met.* The test for pyrogenic substances shall be performed according to the requirements specified in United States Pharmacopeia XX.

(3) *Retest.* If the lot fails to meet the test requirements prescribed in paragraph (b)(2) of this section, the test may be repeated once using five other rabbits. The temperature rises recorded for all eight rabbits used in testing shall be included in determining whether the requirements are met. The lot meets the requirements for absence of pyrogens if not more than three of the eight rabbits show individual rises in temperature of 0.6 °C or more, and if the sum of the eight individual maximum temperature rises does not exceed 3.7 °C.

[38 FR 32056, Nov. 20, 1973, as amended at 40 FR 29710, July 15, 1975; 41 FR 10429, Mar. 11, 1976; 41 FR 41424, Sept. 22, 1976; 44 FR 40289, July 10, 1979; 46 FR 62845, Dec. 29, 1981; 49 FR 15187, Apr. 18, 1984; 50 FR 4134, Jan. 29, 1985; 55 FR 28381, July 11, 1990; 64 FR 56453, Oct. 20, 1999; 67 FR 9587, Mar. 4, 2002; 70 FR 14985, Mar. 24, 2005]

§610.14   Identity.

The contents of a final container of each filling of each lot shall be tested for identity after all labeling operations shall have been completed. The identity test shall be specific for each product in a manner that will adequately identify it as the product designated on final container and package labels and circulars, and distinguish it from any other product being processed in the same laboratory. Identity may be established either through the physical or chemical characteristics of the product, inspection by macroscopic or microscopic methods, specific cultural tests, or in vitro or in vivo immunological tests.

§610.15   Constituent materials.

(a) *Ingredients, preservatives, diluents, adjuvants.* All ingredients used in a licensed product, and any diluent provided as an aid in the administration of the product, shall meet generally accepted standards of purity and quality. Any preservative used shall be sufficiently nontoxic so that the amount present in the recommended dose of the product will not be toxic to the recipient, and in the combination used it shall not denature the specific substances in the product to result in a decrease below the minimum acceptable potency within the dating period when stored at the recommended temperature. Products in multiple-dose containers shall contain a preservative, except that a preservative need not be added to Yellow Fever Vaccine; Poliovirus Vaccine Live Oral; viral vaccines labeled for use with the jet injector; dried vaccines when the accompanying diluent contains a preservative; or to an Allergenic Product in 50 percent or more volume in volume (v/v) glycerin. An adjuvant shall not be introduced into a product unless there is satisfactory evidence that it does not affect adversely the safety or potency of the product. The amount of aluminum in the recommended individual dose of a biological product shall not exceed:

(1) 0.85 milligrams if determined by assay;

(2) 1.14 milligrams if determined by calculation on the basis of the amount of aluminum compound added; or

(3) 1.25 milligrams determined by assay provided that data demonstrating that the amount of aluminum used is safe and necessary to produce the intended effect are submitted to and approved by the Director, Center for Biologics Evaluation and Research or the Director, Center for Drug Evaluation and Research (see mailing addresses in §600.2(a) or (b) of this chapter).

(b) *Extraneous protein; cell culture produced vaccines.* Extraneous protein known to be capable of producing allergenic effects in human subjects shall not be added to a final virus medium of cell culture produced vaccines intended for injection. If serum is used at any stage, its calculated concentration in the final medium shall not exceed 1:1,000,000.

(c) *Antibiotics.* A minimum concentration of antibiotics, other than penicillin, may be added to the production substrate of viral vaccines.

(d) The Director of the Center for Biologics Evaluation and Research or the Director of the Center for Drug Evaluation and Research may approve an exception or alternative to any requirement in this section. Requests for such exceptions or alternatives must be in writing.

[38 FR 32056, Nov. 20, 1973, as amended at 46 FR 51903, Oct. 23, 1981; 48 FR 13025, Mar. 29, 1983; 48 FR 37023, Aug. 16, 1983; 49 FR 23834, June 8, 1984; 50 FR 4134, Jan. 29, 1985; 51 FR 15607, Apr. 25, 1986; 55 FR 11013, Mar. 26, 1990; 70FR 14985, Mar. 24, 2005; 76 FR 20518, Apr. 13, 2011; 80 FR 18093, Apr. 3, 2015]

§610.16   Total solids in serums.

Except as otherwise provided by regulation, no liquid serum or antitoxin shall contain more than 20 percent total solids.

§610.17   Permissible combinations.

Licensed products may not be combined with other licensed products either therapeutic, prophylactic or diagnostic, except as a license is obtained for the combined product. Licensed products may not be combined with nonlicensable therapeutic, prophylactic, or diagnostic substances except as a license is obtained for such combination.

§610.18   Cultures.

(a) *Storage and maintenance.* Cultures used in the manufacture of products shall be stored in a secure and orderly manner, at a temperature and by a method that will retain the initial characteristics of the organisms and insure freedom from contamination and deterioration.

(b) *Identity and verification.* Each culture shall be clearly identified as to source strain. A complete identification of the strain shall be made for each new stock culture preparation. Primary and subsequent seed lots shall be identified by lot number and date of preparation. Periodic tests shall be performed as often as necessary to verify the integrity of the strain characteristics and freedom from extraneous organisms. Results of all periodic tests for verification of cultures and determination of freedom from extraneous organisms shall be recorded and retained.

(c) *Cell lines used for manufacturing biological products*—(1) *General requirements.* Cell lines used for manufacturing biological products shall be:

(i) Identified by history;

(ii) Described with respect to cytogenetic characteristics and tumorigenicity;

(iii) Characterized with respect to in vitro growth characteristics and life potential; and

(iv) Tested for the presence of detectable microbial agents.

(2) *Tests.* Tests that are necessary to assure the safety, purity, and potency of a product may be required by the Director, Center for Biologics Evaluation and Research or the Director, Center for Drug Evaluation and Research.

(3) *Applicability.* This paragraph applies to diploid and nondiploid cell lines. Primary cell cultures that are not subcultivated and primary cell cultures that are subsequently subcultivated for only a very limited number of population doublings are not subject to the provisions of this paragraph (c).

(d) *Records.* The records appropriate for cultures under this section shall be prepared and maintained as required by the applicable provisions of §§211.188 and 211.194 of this chapter.

[38 FR 32056, Nov. 20, 1973, as amended at 51 FR 44453, Dec. 10, 1986; 55 FR 11013, Mar. 26, 1990; 67 FR 9587, Mar. 4, 2002; 70 FR 14985, Mar. 24, 2005]

Subpart C   [Reserved]

§§610.20-610.21   [Reserved]

Subpart D   [Reserved]

§610.30   [Reserved]

Subpart E--Testing Requirements for Relevant Transfusion-Transmitted Infections

§610.39   Definitions.

The definitions set out in §630.3 of this chapter apply to this subpart.
[80 FR 29896, May 22, 2015]

§610.40   Test requirements.

(a) *Human blood and blood components.* Except as specified in paragraphs (c) and (d) of this section, you, an establishment that collects blood and blood components for transfusion or for use in manufacturing a product, including donations intended as a component of, or used to manufacture, a medical device, must comply with the following requirements:

(1) Test each donation for evidence of infection due to the relevant transfusion-transmitted infections described in §630.3(h)(1)(i) through (iii) of this chapter (HIV, HBV, and HCV).

(2) Test each donation for evidence of infection due to the relevant transfusion-transmitted infections described in §630.3(h)(1)(iv) through (vii) of this chapter (HTLV, syphilis, West Nile virus, and Chagas disease). The following exceptions apply:

(i) To identify evidence of infection with syphilis in donors of Source Plasma, you must test donors for evidence of such infection in accordance with §640.65(b) of this chapter, and not under this section.

(ii) You are not required to test donations of Source Plasma for evidence of infection due to the relevant transfusion-transmitted infections described in §630.3(h)(1)(iv), (vi), and (vii) of this chapter (HTLV, West Nile virus, and Chagas disease).

(iii) For each of the relevant transfusion-transmitted infections described in §630.3(h)(1)(iv) through (vii) of this chapter (HTLV, syphilis, West Nile virus, and Chagas disease):

(A) If, based on evidence related to the risk of transmission of that relevant transfusion-transmitted infection, testing each donation is not necessary to reduce adequately and appropriately the risk of transmission of such infection by blood or a blood component, you may adopt an adequate and appropriate alternative testing procedure that has been found acceptable for this purpose by FDA.

(B) If, based on evidence related to the risk of transmission of that relevant transfusion-transmitted infection, testing previously required for that infection is no longer necessary to reduce adequately and appropriately the risk of transmission of such infection by blood or a blood component, you may stop such testing in accordance with procedures found acceptable for this purpose by FDA.

(3) For each of the relevant transfusion-transmitted infections described in §630.3(h)(1)(viii) through (x) of this chapter (CJD, vCJD, malaria) and §630.3(h)(2) of this chapter (other transfusion-transmitted infections):

(i) You must test for evidence of infection when the following conditions are met:

(A) A test(s) for the relevant transfusion-transmitted infection is licensed, approved or cleared by FDA for use as a donor screening test and is available for such use; and

(B) Testing for the relevant transfusion-transmitted infection is necessary to reduce adequately and appropriately the risk of transmission of the relevant transfusion-transmitted infection by blood, or blood component, or blood derivative product manufactured from the collected blood or blood component.

(ii) You must perform this testing on each donation, unless one of the following exceptions applies:

(A) Testing of each donation is not necessary to reduce adequately and appropriately the risk of transmission of such infection by blood, blood component, or blood derivative product manufactured from the collected blood or blood component. When evidence related to the risk of transmission of such infection supports this determination, you may adopt an adequate and appropriate alternative testing procedure that has been found acceptable for this purpose by FDA.

(B) Testing of each donation is not necessary to reduce adequately and appropriately the risk of transmission of such infection by blood, blood component, or blood derivative product manufactured from the collected blood or blood component. When evidence related to the risk of transmission of such infection supports this determination, you may stop such testing in accordance with procedures found acceptable for this purpose by FDA.

(4) Evidence related to the risk of transmission of a relevant transfusion-transmitted infection that would support a determination that testing is not necessary, or that testing of each donation is not necessary, to reduce adequately and appropriately the risk of transmission of such infection by blood or blood component, as described in paragraphs (a)(2)(iii)(A) and (B) of this section, or by blood, blood component, or blood derivative, as described in paragraphs (a)(3)(ii)(A) and (B) of this section, includes epidemiological or other scientific evidence. It may include evidence related to the seasonality or geographic limitation of risk of transmission of such infection by blood or blood component, or other information related to when and how a donation is at risk of transmitting a relevant transfusion-transmitted infection. It may also include evidence related to the effectiveness of manufacturing steps (for example, the use of pathogen reduction technology) that reduce the risk of transmission of the relevant transfusion-transmitted infection by blood, blood components, or blood derivatives, as applicable.

(b) *Testing using one or more licensed, approved, or cleared screening tests.* To perform testing for evidence of infection due to relevant transfusion-transmitted infections as required in paragraph (a) of this section, you must use screening tests that FDA has licensed, approved, or cleared for such use, in accordance with the manufacturer's instructions. You must perform one or more such tests as necessary to reduce adequately and appropriately the risk of transmission of relevant transfusion-transmitted infections.

(c) *Exceptions to testing for dedicated donations, medical devices, and samples.*—(1) Dedicated donations. (i) You must test donations of human blood and blood components from a donor whose donations are dedicated to and used solely by a single identified recipient under paragraphs (a), (b), and (e) of this section; except that, if the donor makes multiple donations for a single identified recipient, you may perform such testing only on the first donation in each 30-day period. If an untested dedicated donation is made available for any use other than transfusion to the single, identified recipient, then this exemption from the testing required under this section no longer applies.

(ii) Each donation must be labeled as required under §606.121 of this chapter and with a label entitled "INTENDED RECIPIENT INFORMATION LABEL" containing the name and identifying information of the recipient. Each donation must also have the following label, as appropriate:

Donor Testing Status	Label
Tests negative	Label as required under §606.121
Tested negative within the last 30 days	"DONOR TESTED WITHIN THE LAST 30 DAYS"

(2) *Source Plasma.* (i) You are not required to test donations of human blood or blood components intended solely as a component of, or used to prepare, a medical device for evidence of infection due to the relevant transfusion-transmitted infections listed in §630.3(h)(iv) of this chapter unless the final device contains viable leukocytes.

(ii) Donations of human blood and blood components intended solely as a component of, or used to prepare, a medical device must be labeled "Caution: For Further Manufacturing Use as a Component of, or to Prepare, a Medical Device."

(3) *Samples.* You are not required to test samples of blood, blood components, plasma, or sera if used or distributed for clinical laboratory testing or research purposes and not intended for administration to humans or in the manufacture of a product.

(d) *Autologous donations.* You, an establishment that collects human blood or blood components from autologous donors, or you, an establishment that is a consignee of a collecting establishment, are not required to test donations of human blood or blood components from autologous donors for evidence of infection due to relevant transfusion-transmitted infections listed in paragraph (a) of this section, except:

(1) If you allow any autologous donation to be used for allogeneic transfusion, you must assure that all autologous donations are tested under this section.

(2) If you ship autologous donations to another establishment that allows autologous donations to be used for allogeneic transfusion, you must assure that all autologous donations shipped to that establishment are tested under this section.

(3) If you ship autologous donations to another establishment that does not allow autologous donations to be used for allogeneic transfusion, you must assure that, at a minimum, the first donation in each 30-day period is tested under this section.

(4) Each autologous donation must be labeled as required under §606.121 of this chapter and with the following label, as appropriate:

Donor Testing Status	Label
Untested	"DONOR UNTESTED"
Tests negative	Label as required under §606.121
Reactive on current collection/reactive in the last 30 days	"BIOHAZARD" legend in §610.40(h)(2)(ii)(B)
Tested negative within the last 30 days	"DONOR TESTED WITHIN THE LAST 30 DAYS"

(e) *Further testing.* You must further test each donation, including autologous donations, found to be reactive by a donor screening test performed under paragraphs (a) and (b) of this section using a licensed, approved, or cleared supplemental test, when available. If no such supplemental test is available, you must perform one or more licensed, approved, or cleared tests as adequate and appropriate to provide additional information concerning the reactive donor's infection status. Except:

(1) For autologous donations:

(i) You must further test under this section, at a minimum, the first reactive donation in each 30 calendar day period; or

(ii) If you have a record for that donor of a positive result on further testing performed under this section, you do not have to further test an autologous donation.

(2) You are not required to perform further testing of a donation found to be reactive by a treponemal donor screening test for syphilis.

(f) *Testing responsibility.* Required testing under this section, must be performed by a laboratory registered in accordance with part 607 of this chapter and either certified to perform such testing on human specimens under the Clinical Laboratory Improvement Amendments of 1988 (42 U.S.C. 263a) under 42 CFR part 493 or has met equivalent requirements as determined by the Centers for Medicare and Medicaid Services in accordance with those provisions.

(g) *Release or shipment prior to testing.* Human blood or blood components that are required to be tested for evidence of infection due to relevant transfusion-transmitted infections designated in paragraph (a) of this section may be released or shipped prior to completion of testing in the following circumstances provided that you label the blood or blood components under §606.121(h) of this chapter, you complete the tests for evidence of infection due to relevant transfusion-transmitted infections as soon as possible after release or shipment, and that you provide the results promptly to the consignee:

(1) Only in appropriately documented medical emergency situations; or

(2) For further manufacturing use as approved in writing by FDA.

(h) *Restrictions on shipment or use*—(1) Reactive screening test. You must not ship or use human blood or blood components that have a reactive screening test for evidence of infection due to relevant transfusion-transmitted infection(s) designated in paragraph (a) of this section or that are collected from a donor with a previous record of a reactive screening test for evidence of infection due to relevant transfusion-transmitted infection(s) designated in paragraph (a) of this section, except as provided in paragraphs (h)(2)(i) through (h)(2)(vii) of this section.

(2) *Exceptions.* (i) You may ship or use blood or blood components intended for autologous use, including reactive donations, as described in paragraph (d) of this section.

(ii) You must not ship or use human blood or blood components that have a reactive screening test for evidence of infection due to a relevant transfusion-transmitted infection(s) designated in paragraph (a) of this section or that are collected from a donor deferred under §610.41(a) unless you meet the following conditions:

(A) Except for autologous donations, you must obtain from FDA written approval for the shipment or use;

(B) You must appropriately label such blood or blood components as required under §606.121 of this chapter, and with the "BIOHAZARD" legend;

(C) Except for autologous donations, you must label such human blood and blood components as reactive for the appropriate screening test for evidence of infection due to the identified relevant transfusion-transmitted infection(s);

(D) If the blood or blood components are intended for further manufacturing use into injectable products, you must include a statement on the container label indicating the exempted use specifically approved by FDA.

(E) Each blood or blood component with a reactive screening test and intended solely as a component of, or used to prepare a medical device, must be labeled with the following label, as appropriate:

Type of Medical Device	Label
A medical device other than an in vitro diagnostic reagent	"Caution: For Further Manufacturing Use as a Component of a Medical Device For Which There Are No AlternativeSources"
An in vitro diagnostic reagent	"Caution: For Further Manufacturing Into In Vitro Diagnostic Reagents For Which There Are No Alternative Sources"

(iii) The restrictions on shipment or use do not apply to samples of blood, blood components, plasma, or sera if used or distributed for clinical laboratory testing or research purposes, and not intended for administration in humans or in the manufacture of a product.

(iv) You may use human blood or blood components from a donor with a previous record of a reactive screening test(s) for evidence of infection due to a relevant transfusion-transmitted infection(s) designated in paragraph (a) of this section, if:

(A) At the time of donation, the donor is shown or was previously shown to be eligible by a requalification method or process found acceptable for such purposes by FDA under §610.41(b); and

(B) tests performed under paragraphs (a) and (b) of this section are nonreactive.

(v) Anti-HBc reactive donations, otherwise nonreactive when tested as required under this section, may be used for further manufacturing into plasma derivatives without prior FDA approval or a "BIOHAZARD" legend as required under paragraphs (h)(2)(ii)(A) and (h)(2)(ii)(B) of this section.

(vi) You may use human blood or blood components, excluding Source Plasma, that test reactive by a screening test for syphilis as required under paragraph (a) of this section if, the donation is further tested by an adequate and appropriate test which demonstrates that the reactive screening test is a biological false positive. You must label the blood or blood components with both test results.

(vii) You may use Source Plasma from a donor who tests reactive by a screening test for syphilis as required under §640.65(a)(2)(ii) and (b)(1)(i) of this chapter, if the donor meets the requirements of §640.65(b)(2)(i) through (b)(2)(iv) of this chapter.

[66 FR 31162, June 11, 2001, as amended at 77 FR 18, Jan. 3, 2012; 80 FR 29896, May 22, 2015]

§610.41   Donor deferral.

(a) You, an establishment that collects human blood or blood components, must defer donors testing reactive by a screening test for evidence of infection due to a relevant transfusion-transmitted infection(s) under §610.40(a), from future donations of human blood and blood components, except:

(1) You are not required to defer a donor who tests reactive for anti-HBc or anti-HTLV, types I and II, on only one occasion. However, you must defer the donor if further testing for HBV or HTLV has been performed under §610.40(e) and the donor is found to be positive, or if a second, licensed, cleared, or approved screening test for HBV or HTLV has been performed on the same donation under §610.40(a) and is reactive, or if the donor tests reactive for anti-HBc or anti-HTLV, types I and II, on more than one occasion;

(2) A deferred donor who tests reactive for evidence of infection due to a relevant transfusion-transmitted infection(s) under §610.40(a) may serve as a donor for blood or blood components shipped or used under §610.40(h) (2)(ii);

(3) A deferred donor who showed evidence of infection due to hepatitis B surface antigen (HBsAg) when previously tested under §610.40(a), (b), and (e) subsequently may donate Source Plasma for use in the preparation of Hepatitis B Immune Globulin (Human) provided the current donation tests nonreactive for HBsAg and the donor is otherwise determined to be eligible;

(4) A deferred donor, who otherwise is determined to be eligible for donation and tests reactive for anti-HBc or for evidence of infection due to HTLV, types I and II, may serve as a donor of Source Plasma;

(5) A deferred donor who tests reactive for a relevant transfusion-transmitted infections(s) under §610.40(a), may serve as an autologous donor under §610.40(d).

(b) A deferred donor subsequently may be found to be eligible as a donor of blood or blood components by a requalification method or process found acceptable for such purposes by FDA. Such a donor is considered no longer deferred.

(c) You must comply with the requirements under §§610.46 and 610.47 when a donor tests reactive by a screening test for HIV or HCV required under §610.40(a) and (b), or when you are aware of other reliable test results or information indicating evidence of HIV or HCV infection.

[66 FR 31164, June 11, 2001, as amended at 72 FR 48798, Aug. 24, 2007; 80 FR 29897, May 22, 2015]

§610.42   Restrictions on use for further manufacture of medical devices.

(a) In addition to labeling requirements in subchapter H of this chapter, when a medical device contains human blood or a blood component as a component of the final device, and the human blood or blood component was found to be reactive by a screening test performed under §610.40(a) and (b), then you must include in the device labeling a statement of warning indicating that the product was manufactured from a donation found to be reactive by a screening test for evidence of infection due to the identified relevant transfusion-transmitted infection(s).

(b) FDA may approve an exception or alternative to the statement of warning required in paragraph (a) of this section based on evidence that the reactivity of the human blood or blood component in the medical device presents no significant health risk through use of the medical device.

[66 FR 31164, June 11, 2001, as amended at 80 FR 29897, May 22, 2015]

§610.44 Use of reference panels by manufacturers of test kits.

(a) When available and appropriate to verify acceptable sensitivity and specificity, you, a manufacturer of test kits, must use a reference panel you obtain from FDA or from an FDA designated source to test lots of the following products. You must test each lot of the following products, unless FDA informs you that less frequent testing is appropriate, based on your consistent prior production of products of acceptable sensitivity and specificity:

(1) A test kit approved for use in testing donations of human blood and blood components for evidence of infection due to relevant transfusion-transmitted infections under §610.40(a); and

(2) Human immunodeficiency virus (HIV) test kit approved for use in the diagnosis, prognosis, or monitoring of this relevant transfusion-transmitted infection.

(b) You must not distribute a lot that is found to be not acceptable for sensitivity and specificity under §610.44(a). FDA may approve an exception or alternative to this requirement. Applicants must submit such requests in writing. However, in limited circumstances, such requests may be made orally and permission may be given orally by FDA. Oral requests and approvals must be promptly followed by written requests and written approvals.

[66 FR 31164, June 11, 2001, as amended at 80 FR 29897, May 22, 2015]

§610.46 Human immunodeficiency virus (HIV) "lookback" requirements.

(a) If you are an establishment that collects Whole Blood or blood components, including Source Plasma and Source Leukocytes, you must establish, maintain, and follow an appropriate system for the following actions:

(1) Within 3 calendar days after a donor tests reactive for evidence of human immunodeficiency virus (HIV) infection when tested under §610.40(a) and (b) or when you are made aware of other reliable test results or information indicating evidence of HIV infection, you must review all

records required under §606.160(d) of this chapter, to identify blood and blood components previously donated by such a donor. For those identified blood and blood components collected:

(i) Twelve months and less before the donor's most recent nonreactive screening tests, or

(ii) Twelve months and less before the donor's reactive direct viral detection test, e.g., nucleic acid test or HIV p24 antigen test, and nonreactive antibody screening test, whichever is the lesser period, you must:

(A) Quarantine all previously collected in-date blood and blood components identified under paragraph (a)(1) of this section if intended for use in another person or for further manufacture into injectable products, except pooled blood components intended solely for further manufacturing into products that are manufactured using validated viral clearance procedures; and

(B) Notify consignees to quarantine all previously collected in-date blood and blood components identified under paragraph (a)(1) of this section if intended for use in another person or for further manufacture into injectable products, except pooled blood components intended solely for further manufacturing into products that are manufactured using validated viral clearance procedures;

(2) You must perform further testing for HIV as required under §610.40(e) of this chapter on the reactive donation.

(3) You must notify consignees of the results of further testing for HIV, or the results of the reactive screening test if further testing under paragraph (a)(2) of this section is not available, or if under an investigational new drug application (IND) or investigational device exemption (IDE), is exempted for such use by FDA, within 45 calendar days after the donor tests reactive for evidence of HIV infection under §610.40(a) and (b) of this chapter. Notification of consignees must include the test results for blood and blood components identified under paragraph (a)(1) of this section that were previously collected from donors who later test reactive for evidence of HIV infection.

(4) You must release from quarantine, destroy, or relabel quarantined in-date blood and blood components, consis-

tent with the results of the further testing performed under paragraph (a)(2) of this section or the results of the reactive screening test if further testing is not available, or if under an IND or IDE, exempted for such use by FDA.

(b) If you are a consignee of Whole Blood or blood components, including Source Plasma and Source Leukocytes, you must establish, maintain, and follow an appropriate system for the following actions:

(1) You must quarantine all previously collected in-date blood and blood components identified under paragraph (a)(1) of this section, except pooled blood components intended solely for further manufacturing into products that are manufactured using validated viral clearance procedures, when notified by the collecting establishment.

(2) You must release from quarantine, destroy, or relabel quarantined in-date blood and blood components consistent with the results of the further testing performed under paragraph (a)(2) of this section, or the results of the reactive screening test if further testing is not available, or if under an IND or IDE, is exempted for such use by FDA.

(3) When further testing for HIV is positive or when the screening test is reactive and further testing is not available, or if under an IND or IDE is exempted for such use by FDA, you must notify transfusion recipients of previous collections of blood and blood components at increased risk of transmitting HIV infection, or the recipient's physician of record, of the need for recipient HIV testing and counseling. You must notify the recipient's physician of record or a legal representative or relative if the recipient is a minor, deceased, adjudged incompetent by a State court, or, if the recipient is competent but State law permits a legal representative or relative to receive information on behalf of the recipient. You must make reasonable attempts to perform the notification within 12 weeks after receiving the results of further testing for evidence of HIV infection from the collecting establishment, or after receiving the donor's reactive screening test result for HIV if further testing is not available, or if under an IND or IDE is exempted for such use by FDA.

(c) Actions under this section do not constitute a recall as defined in §7.3 of this chapter.

[72 FR 48799, Aug. 24, 2007, as amended at 80 FR 29897, May 22, 2015]

§610.47 Hepatitis C virus (HCV)"lookback" requirements.

(a) If you are an establishment that collects Whole Blood or blood components, including Source Plasma and Source Leukocytes, you must establish, maintain, and follow an appropriate system for the following actions:

(1) Within 3 calendar days after a donor tests reactive for evidence of hepatitis C virus (HCV) infection when tested under §610.40(a) and (b) of this chapter or when you are made aware of other reliable test results or information indicating evidence of HCV infection, you must review all records required under §606.160(d) of this chapter, to identify blood and blood components previously donated by such a donor. For those identified blood and blood components collected:

(i) Twelve months and less before the donor's most recent nonreactive screening tests, or

(ii) Twelve months and less before the donor's reactive direct viral detection test, e.g., nucleic acid test and nonreactive antibody screening test, whichever is the lesser period, you must:

(A) Quarantine all previously collected in-date blood and blood components identified under paragraph (a)(1) of this section if intended for use in another person or for further manufacture into injectable products, except pooled blood components intended solely for further manufacturing into products that are manufactured using validated viral clearance procedures; and

(B) Notify consignees to quarantine all previously collected in-date blood and blood components identified under paragraph (a)(1) of this section if intended for use in another person or for further manufacture into injectable products, except pooled blood components intended solely for further manufacturing into products that are manufactured using validated viral clearance procedures;

(2) You must perform further testing for HCV as required under §610.40(e) on the reactive donation.

(3) You must notify consignees of the results of further testing for HCV, or the results of the reactive screening test if further testing is not available, or if under an investigational new drug application (IND) or investigational device exemption (IDE), is exempted for such use by FDA, within 45 calendar days after the donor tests reactive for evidence of HCV infection under §610.40(a) and (b). Notification of consignees must include the test results for blood and blood components identified under paragraph (a)(1) of this section that were previously collected from donors who later test reactive for evidence of HCV infection.

(4) You must release from quarantine, destroy, or relabel quarantined in-date blood and blood components consistent with the results of the further testing performed under paragraph (a)(2) of this section, or the results of the reactive screening test if further testing is not available, or if under an IND or IDE, exempted for such use by FDA.

(b) If you are a consignee of Whole Blood or blood components, including Source Plasma or Source Leukocytes, you must establish, maintain, and follow an appropriate system for the following actions:

(1) You must quarantine all previously collected in-date blood and blood components identified under paragraph (a)(1) of this section, except pooled blood components intended solely for further manufacturing into products that are manufactured using validated viral clearance procedures, when notified by the collecting establishment.

(2) You must release from quarantine, destroy, or relabel quarantined in-date blood and blood components, consistent with the results of the further testing performed under paragraph (a)(2) of this section, or the results of the reactive screening test if further testing is not available, or if under an IND or IDE, is exempted for such use by FDA.

(3) When the further testing for HCV is positive or when the screening test is reactive and further testing is not available, or if under an IND or IDE, is exempted for such

use by FDA, you must notify transfusion recipients of previous collections of blood and blood components at increased risk of transmitting HCV infection, or the recipient's physician of record, of the need for recipient HCV testing and counseling. You must notify the recipient's physician of record or a legal representative or relative if the recipient is a minor, adjudged incompetent by a State court, or if the recipient is competent but State law permits a legal representative or relative to receive information on behalf of the recipient. You must make reasonable attempts to perform the notification within 12 weeks after receiving the results of further testing for evidence of HCV infection from the collecting establishment, or after receiving the donor's reactive screening test result for HCV if further testing is not available, or if under an IND or IDE, is exempted for such use by FDA.

(c) Actions under this section do not constitute a recall as defined in §7.3 of this chapter.

[72 FR 48799, Aug. 24, 2007, as amended at 80 FR 29897, May 22, 2015]

§610.48 [Reserved]

Subpart F--Dating Period Limitations

§610.50 Date of manufacture.

(a) *When the dating period begins.* The dating period for a product must begin on the date of manufacture as described in paragraphs (b) and (c) of this section. The dating period for a combination of two or more products must be no longer than the dating period of the component with the shortest dating period.

(b) *Determining the date of manufacture for biological products other than Whole Blood and blood components.* The date of manufacture for biological products, other than Whole Blood and blood components, must be identified in the approved biologics license application as one of the following, whichever is applicable: The date of:

(1) Potency test or other specific test as described in a biologics license application or supplement to the application;

(2) Removal from animals or humans;

(3) Extraction;

(4) Solution;

(5) Cessation of growth;

(6) Final sterile filtration of a bulk solution;

(7) Manufacture as described in part 660 of this chapter; or

(8) Other specific manufacturing activity described in a biologics license application or supplement to the biologics license application.

(c) *Determining the date of manufacture for Whole Blood and blood components.* (1) The date of manufacture for Whole Blood and blood components must be one of the following, whichever is applicable:

(i) Collection date and/or time;

(ii) Irradiation date;

(iii) The time the red blood cell product was removed from frozen storage for deglycerolization;

(iv) The time the additive or rejuvenation solution was added;

(v) The time the product was entered for washing or removing plasma (if prepared in an open system);

(vi) As specified in the instructions for use by the blood collection, processing, and storage system approved or cleared for such use by FDA; or

(vii) As approved by the Director, Center for Biologics Evaluation and Research, in a biologics license application or supplement to the application.

(2) For licensed Whole Blood and blood components, the date of manufacture must be identified in the approved biologics license application or supplement to the application.

[81 FR 26691, May 4, 2016]

§610.53 Dating periods for licensed biological products.

(a) *General.* Dating periods for Whole Blood and blood components are specified in the table in paragraph (b) of this section.

(b) *Table of dating periods.* In using the table in this paragraph, when a product in column A is stored at the storage temperature prescribed in column B, storage of a product must not exceed the dating period specified in column C, unless a different dating period is specified in the instructions for use by the blood collection, processing and storage system approved or cleared for such use by FDA. Container labels for each product must include the recommended storage temperatures.

Whole Blood and Blood Components Storage Temperatures and Dating Periods

A	B	C
Product	Storage temperature	Dating period
Whole Blood		
ACD, CPD, CP2D	Between 1 and 6 °C	21 days from date of collection.
CPDA-1	do[1]	35 days from date of collection.
Red Blood Cells		
ACD, CPD, CP2D	Between 1 and 6 °C	21 days from date of collection.
CPDA-1	do	35 days from date of collection.
Additive solutions	do	42 days from date of collection.
Open system (e.g., deglycerolized, washed)	do	24 hours after entering bag.
Deglycerolized in closed system with additive solution added	do	14 days after entering bag.
Irradiated	do	28 days from date of irradiation or original dating, whichever is shorter.
Frozen	–65 °C or colder	10 years from date of collection.
Platelets		
Platelets	Between 20 and 24 °C	5 days from date of collection.
Platelets	Other temperatures according to storage bag instructions	As specified in the instructions for use by the blood collection, processing and storage system approved or cleared for such use by the FDA
Plasma		
Fresh Frozen Plasma	–18 °C or colder	1 year from date of collection.
Plasma Frozen Within 24 Hours After Phlebotomy	do	1 year from date of collection.
Plasma Frozen Within 24 Hours After Phlebotomy Held at Room Temperature Up To 24 Hours After Phlebotomy	do	1 year from date of collection.
Plasma Cryoprecipitate Reduced	do	1 year from date of collection.
Plasma	do	5 years from date of collection.
Liquid Plasma	Between 1 and 6 °C	5 days from end of Whole Blood dating period.
Source Plasma (frozen injectable)	–20 °C or colder	10 years from date of collection.
Source Plasma Liquid (injectable)	10 °C or colder	According to approved biologics license application.
Source Plasma (noninjectable)	Temperature appropriate for final product	10 years from date of collection.
Therapeutic Exchange Plasma	–20 °C or colder	10 years from date of collection.
Cryoprecipitated AHF		
Cryoprecipitated AHF	–18 °C or colder	1 year from date of collection of source blood or from date of collection of oldest source blood in pre-storage pool.
Source Leukocytes		
Source Leukocytes	Temperature appropriate for final product	In lieu of expiration date, the collection date must appear on label

1The abbreviation "do." for ditto is used in the table to indicate that the previous line is being repeated.   [81 FR 26691, May 4, 2016]

Subpart G--Labeling Standards
§610.60 Container label.

(a) *Full label*. The following items shall appear on the label affixed to each container of a product capable of bearing a full label:

(1) The proper name of the product;

(2) The name, address, and license number of manufacturer;

(3) The lot number or other lot identification;

(4) The expiration date;

(5) The recommended individual dose, for multiple dose containers.

(6) The statement: "Rx only" for prescription biologicals.

(7) If a Medication Guide is required under part 208 of this chapter, the statement required under §208.24(d) of this chapter instructing the authorized dispenser to provide a Medication Guide to each patient to whom the drug is dispensed and stating how the Medication Guide is provided, except where the container label is too small, the required statement may be placed on the package label.

(b) *Package label information*. If the container is not enclosed in a package, all the items required for a package label shall appear on the container label.

(c) *Partial label*. If the container is capable of bearing only a partial label, the container shall show as a minimum the name (expressed either as the proper or common name), the lot number or other lot identification and the name of the manufacturer; in addition, for multiple dose containers, the recommended individual dose. Containers bearing partial labels shall be placed in a package which bears all the items required for a package label.

(d) *No container label*. If the container is incapable of bearing any label, the items required for a container label may be omitted, provided the container is placed in a package which bears all the items required for a package label.

(e) *Visual inspection*. When the label has been affixed to the container a sufficient area of the container shall remain uncovered for its full length or circumference to permit inspection of the contents.

[38 FR 32056, Nov. 20, 1973, as amended at 47 FR 22518, May 25, 1982; 63 FR 66400, Dec. 1, 1998; 67 FR 4907, Feb. 1, 2002]

§610.61   Package label.

The following items shall appear on the label affixed to each package containing a product:

(a) The proper name of the product;

(b) The name, address, and license number of manufacturer;

(c) The lot number or other lot identification;

(d) The expiration date;

(e) The preservative used and its concentration, or if no preservative is used and the absence of a preservative is a safety factor, the words "no preservative";

(f) The number of containers, if more than one;

(g) The amount of product in the container expressed as (1) the number of doses, (2) volume, (3) units of potency, (4) weight, (5) equivalent volume (for dried product to be reconstituted), or (6) such combination of the foregoing as needed for an accurate description of the contents, whichever is applicable;

(h) The recommended storage temperature;

(i) The words "Shake Well", "Do not Freeze" or the equivalent, as well as other instructions, when indicated by the character of the product;

(j) The recommended individual dose if the enclosed container(s) is a multiple-dose container;

(k) The route of administration recommended, or reference to such directions in an enclosed circular;

(l) Known sensitizing substances, or reference to an enclosed circular containing appropriate information;

(m) The type and calculated amount of antibiotics added during manufacture;

(n) The inactive ingredients when a safety factor, or reference to an enclosed circular containing appropriate information;

(o) The adjuvant, if present;

(p) The source of the product when a factor in safe administration;

(q) The identity of each microorganism used in manufacture, and, where applicable, the production medium and the method of inactivation, or reference to an enclosed circular containing appropriate information;

(r) Minimum potency of product expressed in terms of official standard of potency or, if potency is a factor and no U.S. standard of potency has been prescribed, the words "No U.S. standard of potency."

(s) The statement: "Rx only" for prescription biologicals.

[38 FR 32056, Nov. 20, 1973, as amended at 47 FR 22518, May 25, 1982; 55 FR 10423, Mar. 21, 1990; 67 FR 4907, Feb. 1, 2002]

§610.62   Proper name; package label; legible type.

(a) *Position.* The proper name of the product on the package label shall be placed above any trademark or trade name identifying the product and symmetrically arranged with respect to other printing on the label.

(b) *Prominence.* The point size and typeface of the proper name shall be at least as prominent as the point size and typeface used in designating the trademark and trade name. The contrast in color value between the proper name and the background shall be at least as great as the color value between the trademark and trade name and the background. Typography, layout, contrast, and other printing features shall not be used in a manner that will affect adversely the prominence of the proper name.

(c) *Legible type.* All items required to be on the container label and package label shall be in legible type. "Legible type" is type of a size and character which can be read with ease when held in a good light and with normal vision.

§610.63   Divided manufacturing responsibility to be shown.

If two or more licensed manufacturers participate in the manufacture of a biological product, the name, address, and license number of each must appear on the package label, and on the label of the container if capable of bearing a full label.

[64 FR 56453, Oct. 20, 1999]

§610.64   Name and address of distributor.

The name and address of the distributor of a product may appear on the label provided that the name, address, and license number of the manufacturer also appears on the label and the name of the distributor is qualified by one of the following phrases: "Manufactured for _____", "Distributed by _____", "Manufactured by _____ for _____", "Manufactured for _____ by _____", "Distributor: _____", or "Marketed by _____". The qualifying phrases may be abbreviated.

[61 FR 57330, Nov. 6, 1996]

§610.65   Products for export.

Labels on packages or containers of products for export may be adapted to meet specific requirements of the regulations of the country to which the product is to be exported provided that in all such cases the minimum label requirements prescribed in §610.60 are observed.

§610.67   Bar code label requirements.

Biological products must comply with the bar code requirements at §201.25 of this chapter. However, the bar code requirements do not apply to devices regulated by the Center for Biologics Evaluation and Research or to blood and blood components intended for transfusion. For blood and blood components intended for transfusion, the requirements at §606.121(c)(13) of this chapter apply instead.

[69 FR 9171, Feb. 26, 2004]

§610.68　Exceptions or alternatives to labeling requirements for biological products held by the Strategic National Stockpile.

(a) The appropriate FDA Center Director may grant an exception or alternative to any provision listed in paragraph (f) of this section and not explicitly required by statute, for specified lots, batches, or other units of a biological product, if the Center Director determines that compliance with such labeling requirement could adversely affect the safety, effectiveness, or availability of such product that is or will be included in the Strategic National Stockpile.

(b)(1)(i) A Strategic National Stockpile official or any entity that manufactures (including labeling, packing, relabeling, or repackaging), distributes, or stores a biological product that is or will be included in the Strategic National Stockpile may submit, with written concurrence from a Strategic National Stockpile official, a written request for an exception or alternative described in paragraph (a) of this section to the Center Director.

(ii) The Center Director may grant an exception or alternative described in paragraph (a) of this section on his or her own initiative.

(2) A written request for an exception or alternative described in paragraph (a) of this section must:

(i) Identify the specified lots, batches, or other units of the biological product that would be subject to the exception or alternative;

(ii) Identify the labeling provision(s) listed in paragraph (f) of this section that are the subject of the exception or alternative request;

(iii) Explain why compliance with such labeling provision(s) could adversely affect the safety, effectiveness, or availability of the specified lots, batches, or other units of the biological product that are or will be included in the Strategic National Stockpile;

(iv) Describe any proposed safeguards or conditions that will be implemented so that the labeling of the product includes appropriate information necessary for the safe and effective use of the product, given the anticipated circumstances of use of the product;

(v) Provide a draft of the proposed labeling of the specified lots, batches, or other units of the biological product subject to the exception or alternative; and

(vi) Provide any other information requested by the Center Director in support of the request.

(c) The Center Director must respond in writing to all requests under this section.

(d) A grant of an exception or alternative under this section will include any safeguards or conditions deemed appropriate by the Center Director so that the labeling of product subject to the exception or alternative includes the information necessary for the safe and effective use of the product, given the anticipated circumstances of use.

(e) If you are a sponsor receiving a grant of a request for an exception or alternative to the labeling requirements under this section:

(1) You need not submit a supplement under §601.12(f)(1) through (f)(2) of this chapter; however,

(2) You must report any grant of a request for an exception or alternative under this section as part of your annual report under §601.12(f)(3) of this chapter.

(f) The Center Director may grant an exception or alternative under this section to the following provisions of this chapter, to the extent that the requirements in these provisions are not explicitly required by statute:

(1) §610.60;

(2) §610.61(c) and (e) through (r);

(3) §610.62;

(4) §610.63;

(5) §610.64;

(6) §610.65; and

(7) §312.6.

[72 FR 73600, Dec. 28, 2007]

Notes

Notes

Part 820

The Code of Federal Regulations
Title 21 – Food and Drugs

Part 820
QUALITY SYSTEM REGULATION

Printed by GMP Publications, Inc.
Tel: 866-544-9007 or 856-810-7331
Fax: 866-544-9002
http://www.gmppublications.com
sales@gmppublications.com

PART 820--QUALITY SYSTEM REGULATION

Subpart A--General Provisions

Subpart B--Quality System Requirements

Subpart C--Design Controls

Subpart D--Document Controls

Subpart E--Purchasing Controls

Subpart F--Identification and Traceability

Subpart G--Production and Process Controls

Subpart H--Acceptance Activities

Subpart I--Nonconforming Product

§820.90   Nonconforming product.

Subpart J--Corrective and Preventive Action

§820.100   Corrective and preventive action.

Subpart K--Labeling and Packaging Control

§820.120   Device labeling.
§820.130   Device packaging.

Subpart L--Handling, Storage, Distribution, and Installation

§820.140   Handling.
§820.150   Storage.
§820.160   Distribution.
§820.170   Installation.

Subpart M--Records

§820.180   General requirements.
§820.181   Device master record.
§820.184   Device history record.
§820.186   Quality system record.
§820.198   Complaint files.

Subpart N--Servicing

§820.200   Servicing.

Subpart O--Statistical Techniques

§820.250   Statistical techniques.

Authority: 21 U.S.C. 351, 352, 360, 360c, 360d, 360e, 360h, 360i, 360j, 360l, 371, 374, 381, 383; 42 U.S.C. 216, 262, 263a, 264.

Source: 61 FR 52654, Oct. 7, 1996, unless otherwise noted.

GMP:412020

21 CFR PART 820
QUALITY SYSTEM REGULATION

Subpart A--General Provisions

§820.1   Scope.

(a) *Applicability*.

(1) Current good manufacturing practice (CGMP) requirements are set forth in this quality system regulation. The requirements in this part govern the methods used in, and the facilities and controls used for, the design, manufacture, packaging, labeling, storage, installation, and servicing of all finished devices intended for human use. The requirements in this part are intended to ensure that finished devices will be safe and effective and otherwise in compliance with the Federal Food, Drug, and Cosmetic Act (the act). This part establishes basic requirements applicable to manufacturers of finished medical devices. If a manufacturer engages in only some operations subject to the requirements in this part, and not in others, that manufacturer need only comply with those requirements applicable to the operations in which it is engaged. With respect to class I devices, design controls apply only to those devices listed in §820.30(a)(2). This regulation does not apply to manufacturers of components or parts of finished devices, but such manufacturers are encouraged to use appropriate provisions of this regulation as guidance. Manufacturers of blood and blood components used for transfusion or for further manufacturing are not subject to this part, but are subject to subchapter F of this chapter. Manufacturers of human cells, tissues, and cellular and tissue-based products (HCT/Ps), as defined in §1271.3(d) of this chapter, that are medical devices (subject to premarket review or notification, or exempt from notification, under an application submitted under the device provisions of the act or under a biological product license application under section 351 of the Public Health Service Act) are subject to this part and are also subject to the

donor-eligibility procedures set forth in part 1271 subpart C of this chapter and applicable current good tissue practice procedures in part 1271 subpart D of this chapter. In the event of a conflict between applicable regulations in part 1271 and in other parts of this chapter, the regulation specifically applicable to the device in question shall supersede the more general.

(2) The provisions of this part shall be applicable to any finished device as defined in this part, intended for human use, that is manufactured, imported, or offered for import in any State or Territory of the United States, the District of Columbia, or the Commonwealth of Puerto Rico.

(3) In this regulation the term "where appropriate" is used several times. When a requirement is qualified by "where appropriate," it is deemed to be "appropriate"unless the manufacturer can document justification otherwise. A requirement is "appropriate" if nonimplementation could reasonably be expected to result in the product not meeting its specified requirements or the manufacturer not being able to carry out any necessary corrective action.

(b) The quality system regulation in this part supplements regulations in other parts of this chapter except where explicitly stated otherwise. In the event of a conflict between applicable regulations in this part and in other parts of this chapter, the regulations specifically applicable to the device in question shall supersede any other generally applicable requirements.

(c) *Authority*. Part 820 is established and issued under authority of sections 501, 502, 510, 513, 514, 515, 518, 519, 520, 522, 701, 704, 801, 803 of the act (21 U.S.C. 351, 352, 360, 360c, 360d, 360e, 360h, 360i, 360j, 360l, 371, 374, 381, 383). The failure to comply with any applicable provision in this part renders a device adulterated under section 501(h) of the act. Such a device, as well as any person responsible for the failure to comply, is subject to regulatory action.

(d) *Foreign manufacturers*. If a manufacturer who offers devices for import into the United States refuses to permit or allow the completion of a Food and Drug Administration

(FDA) inspection of the foreign facility for the purpose of determining compliance with this part, it shall appear for purposes of section 801(a) of the act, that the methods used in, and the facilities and controls used for, the design, manufacture, packaging, labeling, storage, installation, or servicing of any devices produced at such facility that are offered for import into the United States do not conform to the requirements of section 520(f) of the act and this part and that the devices manufactured at that facility are adulterated under section 501(h) of the act.

(e) *Exemptions or variances.* (1) Any person who wishes to petition for an exemption or variance from any device quality system requirement is subject to the requirements of section 520(f)(2) of the Federal Food, Drug, and Cosmetic Act. Petitions for an exemption or variance shall be submitted according to the procedures set forth in Sec. 10.30 of this chapter, the FDA's administrative procedures. For guidance on how to proceed for a request for a variance, contact Division of Regulatory Programs 2, Office of Regulatory Programs, Office of Product Evaluation and Quality, Center for Devices and Radiological Health, Food and Drug Administration, 10903 New Hampshire Ave., Bldg. 66, Rm. 1438, Silver Spring, MD 20993-0002.

(2) FDA may initiate and grant a variance from any device quality system requirement when the agency determines that such variance is in the best interest of the public health. Such variance will remain in effect only so long as there remains a public health need for the device and the device would not likely be made sufficiently available without the variance.

[61 FR 52654, Oct. 7, 1996, as amended at 65 FR 17136, Mar. 31, 2000; 65 FR 66636, Nov. 7, 2000; 69 FR 29829, May 25, 2005; 72 FR 17399, Apr. 9, 2007; 75 FR 20915, Apr. 22, 2010; 80 FR 29906, May 22, 2015;85 FR 18442, Apr. 2, 2020]

§820.3   Definitions.

(a) *Act* means the Federal Food, Drug, and Cosmetic Act, as amended (secs. 201-903, 52 Stat. 1040 et seq., as amended (21 U.S.C. 321-394)). All definitions in section 201 of the act shall apply to the regulations in this part.

(b) *Complaint* means any written, electronic, or oral communication that alleges deficiencies related to the identity, quality, durability, reliability, safety, effectiveness, or performance of a device after it is released for distribution.

(c) *Component* means any raw material, substance, piece, part, software, firmware, labeling, or assembly which is intended to be included as part of the finished, packaged, and labeled device.

(d) *Control number* means any distinctive symbols, such as a distinctive combination of letters or numbers, or both, from which the history of the manufacturing, packaging, labeling, and distribution of a unit, lot, or batch of finished devices can be determined.

(e) *Design history file (DHF)* means a compilation of records which describes the design history of a finished device.

(f) *Design input* means the physical and performance requirements of a device that are used as a basis for device design.

(g) *Design output* means the results of a design effort at each design phase and at the end of the total design effort. The finished design output is the basis for the device master record. The total finished design output consists of the device, its packaging and labeling, and the device master record.

(h) *Design review* means a documented, comprehensive, systematic examination of a design to evaluate the adequacy of the design requirements, to evaluate the capability of the design to meet these requirements, and to identify problems.

(i) *Device history record (DHR)* means a compilation of records containing the production history of a finished device.

(j) *Device master record (DMR)* means a compilation of records containing the procedures and specifications for a finished device.

(k) *Establish* means define, document (in writing or electronically), and implement.

(l) *Finished device* means any device or accessory to any device that is suitable for use or capable of functioning, whether or not it is packaged, labeled, or sterilized.

(m) *Lot or batch* means one or more components or finished devices that consist of a single type, model, class, size, composition, or software version that are manufactured under essentially the same conditions and that are intended to have uniform characteristics and quality within specified limits.

(n) *Management with executive responsibility* means those senior employees of a manufacturer who have the authority to establish or make changes to the manufacturer's quality policy and quality system.

(o) *Manufacturer* means any person who designs, manufactures, fabricates, assembles, or processes a finished device. Manufacturer includes but is not limited to those who perform the functions of contract sterilization, installation, relabeling, remanufacturing, repacking, or specification development, and initial distributors of foreign entities performing these functions.

(p) *Manufacturing material* means any material or substance used in or used to facilitate the manufacturing process, a concomitant constituent, or a byproduct constituent produced during the manufacturing process, which is present in or on the finished device as a residue or impurity not by design or intent of the manufacturer.

(q) *Nonconformity* means the nonfulfillment of a specified requirement.

(r) *Product* means components, manufacturing materials, in-process devices, finished devices, and returned devices.

(s) *Quality* means the totality of features and characteristics that bear on the ability of a device to satisfy fitness-for-use, including safety and performance.

(t) *Quality audit* means a systematic, independent examination of a manufacturer's quality system that is performed at defined intervals and at sufficient frequency to determine whether both quality system activities and the results of such activities comply with quality system procedures, that these procedures are implemented effectively, and that these procedures are suitable to achieve quality system objectives.

(u) *Quality policy* means the overall intentions and direction of an organization with respect to quality, as established by management with executive responsibility.

(v) *Quality system* means the organizational structure, responsibilities, procedures, processes, and resources for implementing quality management.

(w) *Remanufacturer* means any person who processes, conditions, renovates, repackages, restores, or does any other act to a finished device that significantly changes the finished device's performance or safety specifications, or intended use.

(x) *Rework* means action taken on a nonconforming product so that it will fulfill the specified DMR requirements before it is released for distribution.

(y) *Specification* means any requirement with which a product, process, service, or other activity must conform.

(z) *Validation* means confirmation by examination and provision of objective evidence that the particular requirements for a specific intended use can be consistently fulfilled.

(1) *Process validation* means establishing by objective evidence that a process consistently produces a result or product meeting its predetermined specifications.

(2) *Design validation* means establishing by objective evidence that device specifications conform with user needs and intended use(s).

(aa) *Verification* means confirmation by examination and provision of objective evidence that specified requirements have been fulfilled.

(bb) *Human cell, tissue, or cellular or tissue-based product (HCT/P) regulated as a device* means an HCT/P as defined in §1271.3(d) of this chapter that does not meet the criteria in §1271.10(a) and that is also regulated as a device.

(cc) *Unique device identifier (UDI)* means an identifier that adequately identifies a device through its distribution and use by meeting the requirements of §830.20 of this chapter. A unique device identifier is composed of:

(1) A *device identifier* - a mandatory, fixed portion of a UDI that identifies the specific version or model of a device and the labeler of that device; and

(2) A *production identifier* - a conditional, variable portion of a UDI that identifies one or more of the following when included on the label of the device:

(i) The lot or batch within which a device was manufactured;

(ii) The serial number of a specific device;

(iii) The expiration date of a specific device;

(iv) The date a specific device was manufactured.

(v) For an HCT/P regulated as a device, the distinct identification code required by §1271.290(c) of this chapter.

(dd) *Universal product code (UPC)* means the product identifier used to identify an item sold at retail in the United States.

[61 FR 52654, Oct. 7, 1996, as amended at 78 FR 55822, Sept. 24, 2013]

§820.5   Quality system.

Each manufacturer shall establish and maintain a quality system that is appropriate for the specific medical device(s) designed or manufactured, and that meets the requirements of this part.

Subpart B--Quality System Requirements

§820.20   Management responsibility.

(a) *Quality policy.* Management with executive responsibility shall establish its policy and objectives for, and commitment to, quality. Management with executive responsibility shall ensure that the quality policy is understood, implemented, and maintained at all levels of the organization.

(b) *Organization.* Each manufacturer shall establish and maintain an adequate organizational structure to ensure that devices are designed and produced in accordance with the requirements of this part.

(1) *Responsibility and authority.* Each manufacturer shall establish the appropriate responsibility, authority, and interrelation of all personnel who manage, perform, and assess work affecting quality, and provide the independence and authority necessary to perform these tasks.

(2) *Resources.* Each manufacturer shall provide adequate resources, including the assignment of trained personnel, for management, performance of work, and assessment activities, including internal quality audits, to meet the requirements of this part.

(3) *Management representative.* Management with executive responsibility shall appoint, and document such appointment of, a member of management who, irrespective of other responsibilities, shall have established authority over and responsibility for:

(i) Ensuring that quality system requirements are effectively established and effectively maintained in accordance with this part; and

(ii) Reporting on the performance of the quality system to management with executive responsibility for review.

(c) *Management review.* Management with executive responsibility shall review the suitability and effectiveness of the quality system at defined intervals and with sufficient frequency according to established procedures to ensure that the quality system satisfies the requirements of this part and the manufacturer's established quality policy and objectives. The dates and results of quality system reviews shall be documented.

(d) *Quality planning.* Each manufacturer shall establish a quality plan which defines the quality practices, resources, and activities relevant to devices that are designed and manufactured. The manufacturer shall establish how the requirements for quality will be met.

(e) *Quality system procedures.* Each manufacturer shall establish quality system procedures and instructions. An outline of the structure of the documentation used in the quality system shall be established where appropriate.

§820.22   Quality audit.

Each manufacturer shall establish procedures for quality audits and conduct such audits to assure that the quality system is in compliance with the established quality system requirements and to determine the effectiveness of the quality system. Quality audits shall be conducted by individuals who do not have direct responsibility for the matters being audited. Corrective action(s), including a reaudit of deficient matters, shall be taken when necessary. A report of the results of each quality audit, and reaudit(s) where taken, shall be made and such reports shall be reviewed by management having responsibility for the matters audited. The dates and results of quality audits and reaudits shall be documented.

§820.25   Personnel.

(a) General. Each manufacturer shall have sufficient personnel with the necessary education, background, training, and experience to assure that all activities required by this part are correctly performed.

(b) Training. Each manufacturer shall establish procedures for identifying training needs and ensure that all personnel are trained to adequately perform their assigned responsibilities. Training shall be documented.

(1) As part of their training, personnel shall be made aware of device defects which may occur from the improper performance of their specific jobs.

(2) Personnel who perform verification and validation activities shall be made aware of defects and errors that may be encountered as part of their job functions.

Subpart C--Design Controls

§820.30 Design controls.

(a) *General.*

(1) Each manufacturer of any class III or class II device, and the class I devices listed in paragraph (a)(2) of this section, shall establish and maintain procedures to control the design of the device in order to ensure that specified design requirements are met.

(2) The following class I devices are subject to design controls:

(i) Devices automated with computer software; and

(ii) The devices listed in the following chart.

Section	Device
868.6810	Catheter, Tracheobronchial Suction.
878.4460	Glove, Surgeon's.
880.6760	Restraint, Protective.
892.5650	System, Applicator, Radionuclide, Manual.
892.5740	Source, Radionuclide Teletherapy.

(b) *Design and development planning.* Each manufacturer shall establish and maintain plans that describe or reference the design and development activities and define responsibility for implementation. The plans shall identify and describe the interfaces with different groups or activities that provide, or result in, input to the design and development process. The plans shall be reviewed, updated, and approved as design and development evolves.

(c) *Design input.* Each manufacturer shall establish and maintain procedures to ensure that the design requirements relating to a device are appropriate and address the intended use of the device, including the needs of the user and patient. The procedures shall include a mechanism for addressing incomplete, ambiguous, or conflicting requirements. The design input requirements shall be documented and shall be reviewed and approved by a designated individual(s). The approval, including the date and signature of the individual(s) approving the requirements, shall be documented.

(d) *Design output.* Each manufacturer shall establish and maintain procedures for defining and documenting design output in terms that allow an adequate evaluation of conformance to design input requirements. Design output procedures shall contain or make reference to acceptance criteria and shall ensure that those design outputs that are essential for the proper functioning of the device are identified. Design output shall be documented, reviewed, and approved before release. The approval, including the date and signature of the individual(s) approving the output, shall be documented.

(e) *Design review.* Each manufacturer shall establish and maintain procedures to ensure that formal documented reviews of the design results are planned and conducted at appropriate stages of the device's design development. The procedures shall ensure that participants at each design review include representatives of all functions concerned with the design stage being reviewed and an individual(s) who does not have direct responsibility for the design stage being reviewed, as well as any specialists needed. The results of a design review, including identification of the design, the date, and the individual(s) performing the review, shall be documented in the design history file (the DHF).

(f) *Design verification.* Each manufacturer shall establish and maintain procedures for verifying the device design. Design verification shall confirm that the design output meets the design input requirements. The results of the design verification, including identification of the design, method(s), the date, and the individual(s) performing the verification, shall be documented in the DHF.

(g) *Design validation.* Each manufacturer shall establish and maintain procedures for validating the device design.

Design validation shall be performed under defined operating conditions on initial production units, lots, or batches, or their equivalents. Design validation shall ensure that devices conform to defined user needs and intended uses and shall include testing of production units under actual or simulated use conditions. Design validation shall include software validation and risk analysis, where appropriate. The results of the design validation, including identification of the design, method(s), the date, and the individual(s) performing the validation, shall be documented in the DHF.

(h) *Design transfer.* Each manufacturer shall establish and maintain procedures to ensure that the device design is correctly translated into production specifications.

(i) *Design changes.* Each manufacturer shall establish and maintain procedures for the identification, documentation, validation or where appropriate verification, review, and approval of design changes before their implementation.

(j) *Design history file.* Each manufacturer shall establish and maintain a DHF for each type of device. The DHF shall contain or reference the records necessary to demonstrate that the design was developed in accordance with the approved design plan and the requirements of this part.

Subpart D--Document Controls

§820.40   Document controls.

Each manufacturer shall establish and maintain procedures to control all documents that are required by this part. The procedures shall provide for the following:

(a) *Document approval and distribution.* Each manufacturer shall designate an individual(s) to review for adequacy and approve prior to issuance all documents established to meet the requirements of this part. The approval, including the date and signature of the individual(s) approving the document, shall be documented. Documents established to meet the requirements of this part shall be available at all locations for which they are designated, used, or otherwise necessary, and all obsolete documents shall be promptly removed from all points of use or otherwise prevented from unintended use.

(b) *Document changes.* Changes to documents shall be reviewed and approved by an individual(s) in the same function or organization that performed the original review and approval, unless specifically designated otherwise. Approved changes shall be communicated to the appropriate personnel in a timely manner. Each manufacturer shall maintain records of changes to documents. Change records shall include a description of the change, identification of the affected documents, the signature of the approving individual(s), the approval date, and when the change becomes effective.

Subpart E--Purchasing Controls

§820.50   Purchasing controls.

Each manufacturer shall establish and maintain procedures to ensure that all purchased or otherwise received product and services conform to specified requirements.

(a) *Evaluation of suppliers, contractors, and consultants.* Each manufacturer shall establish and maintain the requirements, including quality requirements, that must be met by suppliers, contractors, and consultants. Each manufacturer shall:

(1) Evaluate and select potential suppliers, contractors, and consultants on the basis of their ability to meet specified requirements, including quality requirements. The evaluation shall be documented.

(2) Define the type and extent of control to be exercised over the product, services, suppliers, contractors, and consultants, based on the evaluation results.

(3) Establish and maintain records of acceptable suppliers, contractors, and consultants.

(b) *Purchasing data.* Each manufacturer shall establish and maintain data that clearly describe or reference the specified requirements, including quality requirements, for purchased or otherwise received product and services. Purchasing documents shall include, where possible, an agreement that the suppliers, contractors, and consultants agree to notify the manufacturer of changes in the product or service so that manufacturers may determine whether the changes may affect the quality of a finished device. Purchasing data shall be approved in accordance with §820.40.

Subpart F--Identification and Traceability

§820.60   Identification.

Each manufacturer shall establish and maintain procedures for identifying product during all stages of receipt, production, distribution, and installation to prevent mixups.

§820.65   Traceability.

Each manufacturer of a device that is intended for surgical implant into the body or to support or sustain life and whose failure to perform when properly used in accordance with instructions for use provided in the labeling can be reasonably expected to result in a significant injury to the user shall establish and maintain procedures for identitylng with a control number each unit, lot, or batch of finished devices and where approprlate components. The procedures shall facilitate corrective action. Such identification shall be documented in the DHR.

Subpart G--Production and Process Controls

§820.70   Production and process controls.

(a) *General.* Each manufacturer shall develop, conduct, control, and monitor production processes to ensure that a device conforms to its specifications. Where deviations from device specifications could occur as a result of the manufacturing process, the manufacturer shall establish and maintain process control procedures that describe any process controls necessary to ensure conformance to specifications. Where process controls are needed they shall include:

(1) Documented instructions, standard operating procedures (SOP's), and methods that define and control the manner of production;

(2) Monitoring and control of process parameters and component and device characteristics during production;

(3) Compliance with specified reference standards or codes;

(4) The approval of processes and process equipment; and

(5) Criteria for workmanship which shall be expressed in documented standards or by means of identified and approved representative samples.

(b) *Production and process changes.* Each manufacturer shall establish and maintain procedures for changes to a specification, method, process, or procedure. Such changes shall be verified or where appropriate validated according to §820.75, before implementation and these activities shall be documented. Changes shall be approved in accordance with §820.40.

(c) *Environmental control.* Where environmental conditions could reasonably be expected to have an adverse effect on product quality, the manufacturer shall establish and maintain procedures to adequately control these environmental conditions. Environmental control system(s) shall be periodically inspected to verify that the system, including necessary equipment, is adequate and functioning properly. These activities shall be documented and reviewed.

(d) *Personnel.* Each manufacturer shall establish and maintain requirements for the health, cleanliness, personal practices, and clothing of personnel if contact between such personnel and product or environment could reasonably be expected to have an adverse effect on product quality. The manufacturer shall ensure that maintenance and other personnel who are required to work temporarily under special environmental conditions are appropriately trained or supervised by a trained individual.

(e) *Contamination control.* Each manufacturer shall establish and maintain procedures to prevent contamination of equipment or product by substances that could reasonably be expected to have an adverse effect on product quality.

(f) *Buildings.* Buildings shall be of suitable design and contain sufficient space to perform necessary operations, prevent mixups, and assure orderly handling.

(g) *Equipment.* Each manufacturer shall ensure that all equipment used in the manufacturing process meets specified requirements and is appropriately designed, constructed, placed, and installed to facilitate maintenance, adjustment, cleaning, and use.

(1) *Maintenance schedule.* Each manufacturer shall establish and maintain schedules for the adjustment, cleaning, and other maintenance of equipment to ensure that manufacturing specifications are met. Maintenance activities, including the date and individual(s) performing the maintenance activities, shall be documented.

(2) *Inspection.* Each manufacturer shall conduct periodic inspections in accordance with established procedures to ensure adherence to applicable equipment maintenance schedules. The inspections, including the date and individual(s) conducting the inspections, shall be documented.

(3) *Adjustment.* Each manufacturer shall ensure that any inherent limitations or allowable tolerances are visibly posted on or near equipment requiring periodic adjustments or are readily available to personnel performing these adjustments.

(h) *Manufacturing material.* Where a manufacturing material could reasonably be expected to have an adverse effect on product quality, the manufacturer shall establish and maintain procedures for the use and removal of such manufacturing material to ensure that it is removed or limited to an amount that does not adversely affect the device's quality. The removal or reduction of such manufacturing material shall be documented.

(i) *Automated processes.* When computers or automated data processing systems are used as part of production or the quality system, the manufacturer shall validate computer software for its intended use according to an established protocol. All software changes shall be validated before approval and issuance. These validation activities and results shall be documented.

§820.72 Inspection, measuring, and test equipment.

(a) *Control of inspection, measuring, and test equipment.* Each manufacturer shall ensure that all inspection, measuring, and test equipment, including mechanical, automated, or electronic inspection and test equipment, is suitable for its intended purposes and is capable of producing valid results. Each manufacturer shall establish and maintain procedures to ensure that equipment is routinely calibrated, inspected, checked, and maintained. The procedures shall include provisions for handling, preservation, and storage of equipment, so that its accuracy and fitness for use are maintained. These activities shall be documented.

(b) *Calibration.* Calibration procedures shall include specific directions and limits for accuracy and precision. When accuracy and precision limits are not met, there shall be provisions for remedial action to reestablish the limits and to evaluate whether there was any adverse effect on the device's quality. These activities shall be documented.

(1) *Calibration standards.* Calibration standards used for inspection, measuring, and test equipment shall be traceable to national or international standards. If national or international standards are not practical or available, the manufacturer shall use an independent reproducible standard. If no applicable standard exists, the manufacturer shall establish and maintain an in-house standard.

(2) *Calibration records.* The equipment identification, calibration dates, the individual performing each calibration, and the next calibration date shall be documented. These records shall be displayed on or near each piece of equipment or shall be readily available to the personnel using such equipment and to the individuals responsible for calibrating the equipment.

§820.75   Process validation.

(a) Where the results of a process cannot be fully verified by subsequent inspection and test, the process shall be validated with a high degree of assurance and approved according to established procedures. The validation activities and results, including the date and signature of the individual(s) approving the validation and where appropriate the major equipment validated, shall be documented.

(b) Each manufacturer shall establish and maintain procedures for monitoring and control of process parameters for validated processes to ensure that the specified requirements continue to be met.

(1) Each manufacturer shall ensure that validated processes are performed by qualified individual(s).

(2) For validated processes, the monitoring and control methods and data, the date performed, and, where appropriate, the individual(s) performing the process or the major equipment used shall be documented.

(c) When changes or process deviations occur, the manufacturer shall review and evaluate the process and perform revalidation where appropriate. These activities shall be documented.

Subpart H--Acceptance Activities

§820.80   Receiving, in-process, and finished device acceptance.

(a) *General.* Each manufacturer shall establish and maintain procedures for acceptance activities. Acceptance activities include inspections, tests, or other verification activities.

(b) *Receiving acceptance activities.* Each manufacturer shall establish and maintain procedures for acceptance of incoming product. Incoming product shall be inspected, tested, or otherwise verified as conforming to specified requirements. Acceptance or rejection shall be documented.

(c) *In-process acceptance activities.* Each manufacturer shall establish and maintain acceptance procedures, where appropriate, to ensure that specified requirements for in-process product are met. Such procedures shall ensure that in-process product is controlled until the required inspection and tests or other verification activities have been completed, or necessary approvals are received, and are documented.

(d) *Final acceptance activities.* Each manufacturer shall establish and maintain procedures for finished device acceptance to ensure that each production run, lot, or batch of finished devices meets acceptance criteria. Finished devices shall be held in quarantine or otherwise adequately controlled until released. Finished devices shall not be released for distribution until:

(1) The activities required in the DMR are completed;

(2) the associated data and documentation is reviewed;

(3) the release is authorized by the signature of a designated individual(s); and

(4) the authorization is dated.

(e) *Acceptance records.* Each manufacturer shall document acceptance activities required by this part. These records shall include:

(1) The acceptance activities performed;

(2) the dates acceptance activities are performed;

(3) the results;

(4) the signature of the individual(s) conducting the acceptance activities; and

(5) where appropriate the equipment used. These records shall be part of the DHR.

§820.86   Acceptance status.

Each manufacturer shall identify by suitable means the acceptance status of product, to indicate the conformance or nonconformance of product with acceptance criteria. The identification of acceptance status shall be maintained throughout manufacturing, packaging, labeling, installation, and servicing of the product to ensure that only product which has passed the required acceptance activities is distributed, used, or installed.

Subpart I--Nonconforming Product

§820.90 Nonconforming product.

(a) *Control of nonconforming product.* Each manufacturer shall establish and maintain procedures to control product that does not conform to specified requirements. The procedures shall address the identification, documentation, evaluation, segregation, and disposition of nonconforming product. The evaluation of nonconformance shall include a determination of the need for an investigation and notification of the persons or organizations responsible for the nonconformance. The evaluation and any investigation shall be documented.

(b) *Nonconformity review and disposition.*

(1) Each manufacturer shall establish and maintain procedures that define the responsibility for review and the authority for the disposition of nonconforming product. The procedures shall set forth the review and disposition process. Disposition of nonconforming product shall be documented. Documentation shall include the justification for use of nonconforming product and the signature of the individual(s) authorizing the use.

(2) Each manufacturer shall establish and maintain procedures for rework, to include retesting and reevaluation of the nonconforming product after rework, to ensure that the product meets its current approved specifications. Rework and reevaluation activities, including a determination of any adverse effect from the rework upon the product, shall be documented in the DHR.

Subpart J--Corrective and Preventive Action

§820.100 Corrective and preventive action.

(a) Each manufacturer shall establish and maintain procedures for implementing corrective and preventive action. The procedures shall include requirements for:

(1) Analyzing processes, work operations, concessions, quality audit reports, quality records, service records, complaints, returned product, and other sources of quality

data to identify existing and potential causes of nonconforming product, or other quality problems. Appropriate statistical methodology shall be employed where necessary to detect recurring quality problems;

(2) Investigating the cause of nonconformities relating to product, processes, and the quality system;

(3) Identifying the action(s) needed to correct and prevent recurrence of nonconforming product and other quality problems;

(4) Verifying or validating the corrective and preventive action to ensure that such action is effective and does not adversely affect the finished device;

(5) Implementing and recording changes in methods and procedures needed to correct and prevent identified quality problems;

(6) Ensuring that information related to quality problems or nonconforming product is disseminated to those directly responsible for assuring the quality of such product or the prevention of such problems; and

(7) Submitting relevant information on identified quality problems, as well as corrective and preventive actions, for management review.

(b) All activities required under this section, and their results, shall be documented.

Subpart K--Labeling and Packaging Control

§820.120   Device labeling.

Each manufacturer shall establish and maintain procedures to control labeling activities.

(a) *Label integrity.* Labels shall be printed and applied so as to remain legible and affixed during the customary conditions of processing, storage, handling, distribution, and where appropriate use.

(b) *Labeling inspection.* Labeling shall not be released for storage or use until a designated individual(s) has examined the labeling for accuracy including, where applicable, the correct unique device identifier (UDI) or universal product code (UPC), expiration date, control number, storage instructions, handling instructions, and any additional processing instructions. The release, including the date and signature of the individual(s) performing the examination, shall be documented in the DHR.

(c) *Labeling storage.* Each manufacturer shall store labeling in a manner that provides proper identification and is designed to prevent mixups.

(d) *Labeling operations.* Each manufacturer shall control labeling and packaging operations to prevent labeling mixups. The label and labeling used for each production unit, lot, or batch shall be documented in the DHR.

(e) *Control number.* Where a control number is required by §820.65, that control number shall be on or shall accompany the device through distribution.

[61 FR 52654, Oct. 7, 1996, as amended at 78 FR 55822, Sept. 24, 2013]

§820.130   Device packaging.

Each manufacturer shall ensure that device packaging and shipping containers are designed and constructed to protect the device from alteration or damage during the customary conditions of processing, storage, handling, and distribution.

Subpart L--Handling, Storage, Distribution, and Installation

§820.140   Handling.

Each manufacturer shall establish and maintain procedures to ensure that mixups, damage, deterioration, contamination, or other adverse effects to product do not occur during handling.

§820.150   Storage.

(a) Each manufacturer shall establish and maintain procedures for the control of storage areas and stock rooms for product to prevent mixups, damage, deterioration, contamination, or other adverse effects pending use or distribution and to ensure that no obsolete, rejected, or deteriorated product is used or distributed. When the quality of product deteriorates over time, it shall be stored in a manner to facilitate proper stock rotation, and its condition shall be assessed as appropriate.

(b) Each manufacturer shall establish and maintain procedures that describe the methods for authorizing receipt from and dispatch to storage areas and stock rooms.

§820.160   Distribution.

(a) Each manufacturer shall establish and maintain procedures for control and distribution of finished devices to ensure that only those devices approved for release are distributed and that purchase orders are reviewed to ensure that ambiguities and errors are resolved before devices are released for distribution. Where a device's fitness for use or quality deteriorates over time, the procedures shall ensure that expired devices or devices deteriorated beyond acceptable fitness for use are not distributed.

(b) Each manufacturer shall maintain distribution records which include or refer to the location of:

(1) The name and address of the initial consignee;

(2) The identification and quantity of devices shipped;

(3) The date shipped; and

(4) Any control number(s) used.

§820.170   Installation.

(a) Each manufacturer of a device requiring installation shall establish and maintain adequate installation and inspection instructions, and where appropriate test procedures. Instructions and procedures shall include directions for ensuring proper installation so that the device will perform as intended after installation. The manufacturer shall distribute the instructions and procedures with the device or otherwise make them available to the person(s) installing the device.

(b) The person installing the device shall ensure that the installation, inspection, and any required testing are performed in accordance with the manufacturer's instructions and procedures and shall document the inspection and any test results to demonstrate proper installation.

Subpart M--Records

§820.180   General requirements.

All records required by this part shall be maintained at the manufacturing establishment or other location that is reasonably accessible to responsible officials of the manufacturer and to employees of FDA designated to perform inspections. Such records, including those not stored at the inspected establishment, shall be made readily available for review and copying by FDA employee(s). Such records shall be legible and shall be stored to minimize deterioration and to prevent loss. Those records stored in automated data processing systems shall be backed up.

(a) *Confidentiality*. Records deemed confidential by the manufacturer may be marked to aid FDA in determining whether information may be disclosed under the public information regulation in part 20 of this chapter.

(b) *Record retention period*. All records required by this part shall be retained for a period of time equivalent to the design and expected life of the device, but in no case less than 2 years from the date of release for commercial distribution by the manufacturer.

(c) *Exceptions*. This section does not apply to the reports required by §820.20(c) Management review, §820.22 Quality audits, and supplier audit reports used to meet the requirements of §820.50(a) Evaluation of suppliers, contractors, and consultants, but does apply to procedures established under these provisions. Upon request of a designated employee of FDA, an employee in management with executive responsibility shall certify in writing that the management reviews and quality audits required under this part, and supplier audits where applicable, have been performed and documented, the dates on which they were performed, and that any required corrective action has been undertaken.

§820.181   Device master record.

Each manufacturer shall maintain device master records (DMR's). Each manufacturer shall ensure that each DMR is prepared and approved in accordance with §820.40. The DMR for each type of device shall include, or refer to the location of, the following information:

(a) Device specifications including appropriate drawings, composition, formulation, component specifications, and software specifications;

(b) Production process specifications including the appropriate equipment specifications, production methods, production procedures, and production environment specifications;

(c) Quality assurance procedures and specifications including acceptance criteria and the quality assurance equipment to be used;

(d) Packaging and labeling specifications, including methods and processes used; and

(e) Installation, maintenance, and servicing procedures and methods.

§820.184   Device history record.

Each manufacturer shall maintain device history records (DHR's). Each manufacturer shall establish and maintain procedures to ensure that DHR's for each batch, lot, or unit are maintained to demonstrate that the device is manufactured in accordance with the DMR and the requirements of this part. The DHR shall include, or refer to the location of, the following information:

(a) The dates of manufacture;

(b) The quantity manufactured;

(c) The quantity released for distribution;

(d) The acceptance records which demonstrate the device is manufactured in accordance with the DMR;

(e) The primary identification label and labeling used for each production unit; and

(f) Any unique device identifier (UDI) or universal product code (UPC), and any other device identification(s) and control number(s) used.

[61 FR 52654, Oct. 7, 1996, as amended at 78 FR 55822, Sept. 24, 2013]

§820.186   Quality system record.

Each manufacturer shall maintain a quality system record (QSR). The QSR shall include, or refer to the location of, procedures and the documentation of activities required by this part that are not specific to a particular type of device(s), including, but not limited to, the records required by §820.20. Each manufacturer shall ensure that the QSR is prepared and approved in accordance with §820.40.

§820.198   Complaint files.

(a) Each manufacturer shall maintain complaint files. Each manufacturer shall establish and maintain procedures for receiving, reviewing, and evaluating complaints by a formally designated unit. Such procedures shall ensure that:

(1) All complaints are processed in a uniform and timely manner;

(2) Oral complaints are documented upon receipt; and

(3) Complaints are evaluated to determine whether the complaint represents an event which is required to be reported to FDA under part 803 of this chapter, Medical Device Reporting.

(b) Each manufacturer shall review and evaluate all complaints to determine whether an investigation is necessary. When no investigation is made, the manufacturer shall maintain a record that includes the reason no investigation was made and the name of the individual responsible for the decision not to investigate.

(c) Any complaint involving the possible failure of a device, labeling, or packaging to meet any of its specifications shall be reviewed, evaluated, and investigated, unless such investigation has already been performed for a similar complaint and another investigation is not necessary.

(d) Any complaint that represents an event which must be reported to FDA under part 803 of this chapter shall be promptly reviewed, evaluated, and investigated by a designated individual(s) and shall be maintained in a separate portion of the complaint files or otherwise clearly identified. In addition to the information required by §820.198(e), records of investigation under this paragraph shall include a determination of:

(1) Whether the device failed to meet specifications;

(2) Whether the device was being used for treatment or diagnosis; and

(3) The relationship, if any, of the device to the reported incident or adverse event.

(e) When an investigation is made under this section, a record of the investigation shall be maintained by the formally designated unit identified in paragraph (a) of this section. The record of investigation shall include:

(1) The name of the device;

(2) The date the complaint was received;

(3) Any unique device identifier (UDI) or universal product code (UPC), and any other device identification(s) and control number(s) used;

(4) The name, address, and phone number of the complainant;

(5) The nature and details of the complaint;

(6) The dates and results of the investigation;

(7) Any corrective action taken; and

(8) Any reply to the complainant.

(f) When the manufacturer's formally designated complaint unit is located at a site separate from the manufacturing establishment, the investigated complaint(s) and the record(s) of investigation shall be reasonably accessible to the manufacturing establishment.

(g) If a manufacturer's formally designated complaint unit is located outside of the United States, records required by this section shall be reasonably accessible in the United States at either:

(1) A location in the United States where the manufacturer's records are regularly kept; or

(2) The location of the initial distributor.

[61 FR 52654, Oct. 7, 1996, as amended at 69 FR 11313, Mar. 10, 2004; 71 FR 16228, Mar. 31, 2006; 78 FR 55822, Sept. 24, 2013]

Subpart N--Servicing

§820.200 Servicing.

(a) Where servicing is a specified requirement, each manufacturer shall establish and maintain instructions and procedures for performing and verifying that the servicing meets the specified requirements.

(b) Each manufacturer shall analyze service reports with appropriate statistical methodology in accordance with §820.100.

(c) Each manufacturer who receives a service report that represents an event which must be reported to FDA under part 803 of this chapter shall automatically consider the report a complaint and shall process it in accordance with the requirements of §820.198.

(d) Service reports shall be documented and shall include:

(1) The name of the device serviced;

(2) Any unique device identifier (UDI) or universal product code (UPC), and any other device identification(s) and control number(s) used;

(3) The date of service;

(4) The individual(s) servicing the device;

(5) The service performed; and

(6) The test and inspection data.

[61 FR 52654, Oct. 7, 1996, as amended at 69 FR 11313, Mar. 10, 2004; 78 FR 55822, Sept. 24, 2013]

Subpart O--Statistical Techniques

§820.250 Statistical techniques.

(a) Where appropriate, each manufacturer shall establish and maintain procedures for identifying valid statistical techniques required for establishing, controlling, and verifying the acceptability of process capability and product characteristics.

(b) Sampling plans, when used, shall be written and based on a valid statistical rationale. Each manufacturer shall establish and maintain procedures to ensure that sampling methods are adequate for their intended use and to ensure that when changes occur the sampling plans are reviewed. These activities shall be documented.

Notes

Notes

Notes